M000210053

FROM MAC AND CHEESE TO VEGGIES PLEASE

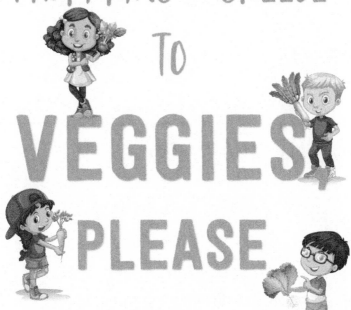

How to get your kid to eat new foods, end picky eating forever, and stay sane in the process.

JENNIFER SCRIBNER, NTP

Copyright © 2017 by JENNIFER SCRIBNER.
All rights reserved. This book or any portion thereof may not be reproduced or used in any manner whatsoever without the express written permission of the publisher except for the use of brief quotations in a book review.

Publishing Services provided by Paper Raven Books
Printed in the United States of America
First Printing, 2017

ISBN
Paperback = 978-0-9997101-0-4
Hardback = 978-0-9997101-1-1

TABLE OF CONTENTS

To the moms who taught me that determination is the most important trait in overcoming picky eating. Thank you for experimenting with me.

To my husband, Seth. Your consistent encouragement and faith in me is the reason this book is complete. You were right.

And to my dear sweet kitty, Uke, who passed away just before publication. It was easy to love the hours spent writing, with you on my lap. You were the best co-worker ever.

INTRODUCTION

Imagine it's a pleasant spring evening and your kids are in the backyard barefoot, playing on the grass together. You're in the kitchen taking a pot roast from the slow cooker and dishing it up on plates along with cooked vegetables like broccoli, onions, Brussels sprouts, carrots, celery, and zucchini. Everyone gets a couple tablespoons of homemade sauerkraut and a mug of broth to drink. When you call the kids, they all run in happily, sit down at the table, put a napkin on their lap, and start eating with no complaints.

If this dinner time is just a fantasy for you, consider this a glimpse into your future.

Your child's illnesses, rashes, stomach aches, and behavioral issues finally have an answer. It's something in their diet that needs to change, and yet making that change can feel like a monumental undertaking. This is especially true if your kid is a picky eater, which is so common now that many people consider it normal. It doesn't have to be that way.

Right now, you're sick of having these food fights with your kids. You're tired of feeling guilty about letting this pickiness go on too long. You're embarrassed about the behavior issues, taking too many sick days, or not following the recommendations you've been given by your healthcare practitioner.

You also likely have other children or household members who don't need a special diet. And you have your hands full with your normal, everyday tasks. How will you find time to add yet another thing to your full plate? Are you going to end up making different meals for everyone in the house, or can you get everyone on board to eat the same thing? Where do you start with this big change? And where can you turn if you run into problems and have questions?

Making a big food change with your picky eater isn't going to be easy at first, but the strategies and tips in this book will set you on the course for your dream life in the future. Instead of dinner being a stressful fight, you can breathe a sigh of relief as you serve your children nutritious foods that they'll eat happily every day.

Sorting through the dietary advice and choosing the healing approach that seems right for your child is one thing, but implementing it with your kid is where the real work begins. The needed foods and cooking alone take some learning, planning, and effort. I'm here to show you how to implement the healing diet you've chosen in the toughest situation—with your picky eater.

In this book, you'll learn:

- How our modern food, medicine, and everyday toxin exposures have left you with a kid who's picky and unhealthy.

- How to set goals for your child's healing, gather support from those around you (or get support elsewhere), and prioritize budget choices.

- Three methods to get your child on a new healing diet, with recommendations for different age groups.

- General principles of healing and repopulating the digestive system, which are common in most healing diets.

- What to expect during the first two weeks, which is the toughest time.

- Supplements and foods that can accelerate healing.

- When and how to build in daily detoxification strategies.

- Troubleshooting tips for the most common problems you'll encounter, like constipation, bedwetting, and eczema.

- What to do if you get stuck and want to give up.

- Plus, a section on alternatives if you find your child won't eat or drink something that's required on the diet you've chosen.

On the flip-side, here's what you won't learn in this book:

- Healing advice for particular illnesses. I trust you've investigated that already and that's how you came to decide a special diet was necessary.

- The philosophy of any one diet. I will mention a few foods that are common to many healing diets, which may or may not be applicable to the one you're using.

- Recipes and cooking techniques.

- Health or picky eating in adults.

- How to come off of your chosen diet when healing is complete.

- How to take your child off of any medications. Please consult your pediatrician to help you with those.

This book has strategies for you, whether you're switching to gluten-free/casein-free (GF/CF), sugar-free, Weston A. Price, the Gut and Psychology Syndrome (GAPS) Diet, Feingold, Specific Carbohydrate Diet (SCD), Paleo, Body Ecology Diet, or just an elimination diet.

Most therapeutic healing diets aren't intended to be followed forever, but the length of time you follow them depends on how quickly your child heals. You won't ever go back to eating a diet filled with convenience foods, but I promise you won't want to. Once you've stripped the processed foods and preservatives off your kids' taste buds, they'll prefer nutritious foods. Healing diets are all based on whole foods, so much of what you incorporate will be commonplace in the long run, with the freedom to expand out of a strict food list.

From Mac & Cheese to Veggies, Please shows you how to get your child eating their new diet without a constant fight. It's not one single prescribed path, because every child is different, and different parents are comfortable trialing different strategies. I've created *From Mac & Cheese to Veggies, Please* to highlight strategies and overcome sticking points, so you can get *your* picky kids eating only these new foods within weeks. Then, you'll begin to see the *real* results: fewer colds, coughs, and tummy aches, less food sensitivity, better focus, easy sleep, quicker language development, and better emotional regulation.

Remember that "fantasy" at the beginning of the book about the family sitting down to eat a nutritious meal happily with no complaints? It's not just a fantasy. It's within your reach. I'll show you how to get there.

PREFACE

I was a picky eater well into adulthood. I was in my 30s and sick and tired of my daily acne breakouts. I'd spent thousands of dollars on designer skin care and dermatologists, and it was *still* a problem.

I realized there had to be something going on inside my body that was showing up on my face, and I was determined to figure out what it was. I read every skin health book and study I could find, and used that information to create my own "diet" to follow for three months. I gave up processed foods and vegetarianism, and focused on nutrient-dense whole foods like my grandparents ate growing up. Not only did my skin clear, but I had more energy than ever and needed less sleep.

At the end of those three months, I stumbled upon an advertisement for the Nutritional Therapy Association, and it turned out that their program taught the things I had just learned about myself! It was that bolt-of-lightening moment where I just felt this was the next step, even though I didn't know where that path would take me.

I heard about the success of the GAPS Diet in 2010 when I was studying at the Nutritional Therapy Association. When Dr. Natasha Campbell-McBride, creator of the GAPS Nutritional Program and author of *Gut and Psychology Syndrome*, announced her first Practitioner Training in the U.S., I jumped at the chance to attend.

In September 2011, I had freshly graduated from the Nutritional Therapy Program and was hungry to learn even more. I wanted to try the GAPS Diet myself but didn't dare commit to something so intense while I was still in school and also working full-time. Our household began the GAPS Intro Diet in October 2011 (right after my birthday, so I didn't miss out on cake). Even though I started from a pretty healthy place by that point, my energy, mental clarity, and sugar cravings all improved dramatically. You can read my full GAPS Intro Diet diary on my website.

Being one of the first Certified GAPS Diet Practitioners in the United States meant that I soon started getting calls from people who needed help getting started with, or troubleshooting issues on, the GAPS Diet. Experience was my best teacher, and I'm not someone who shies away from complicated cases. I welcomed all kinds of GAPS people into my private practice and group classes. Within months, I was working exclusively with the GAPS Diet, and that's what I did for the following six years.

I've followed the work of several physicians and researchers, with Dr. Campbell McBride being the most prominent in my life. I'm indebted to her for helping me understand how the gut connects to the whole body and the brain, as well as all the factors that converge to turn our kids into picky eaters. (If you'd like more information about GAPS, please see the *Resources* section).

Over the past several years, I've learned so much from my clients in developing a system to help them get prepared for a dramatic diet change, along with strategies to help them succeed. I'm a person who naturally thinks step-by-step while keeping my sights on the big picture. I have a vast amount of knowledge, but I don't have the magic answer for anyone. Each person on earth is a unique individual, so I help people customize their diet to each member of their family. I can see what's most likely going to work, but we go forward like it's a science experiment: trialing something, gathering the results, and tweaking it to make it better.

In *From Mac & Cheese to Veggies, Please,* I'm sharing the processes I use with my one-on-one clients to get their picky kids on a dramatically different diet quickly, plus all kinds of customizing and troubleshooting resources. By the end of this book, you'll have the knowledge and advice you need to get great results with your own healing diet experiment.

You'll read some of my success stories throughout this book, and I'd love to hear yours when you've used this guide to help you implement a new healing diet with your picky kids!

Share your success story with me through the *Contact* page on my website: www.bodywisdomnutrition.com.

CHAPTER 1: HOW YOU GOT A PICKY KID

A success story is the first thing most of us hear about a healing diet. When you come across one that describes you or your family's health problem being healed, it's incredibly motivating. So, what's the next thing that people do? Look up what they can and can't eat on that diet and how to get started. There's actually a step in between there, and I want to make sure you don't miss it. We're going back to the basics of how your kid developed into their illness in the first place, and how changing their diet will heal them.

A certain combination of toxicity, diet, and lifestyle issues come together in different ways to create today's sick kids. Understanding how your kid came to be this way, and how therapeutic diets work to reverse their symptoms, will help you stick with the diet through the tough times. This book is about action, with strategies and tips for getting your kids eating. But let's start with a refresher on how most illnesses begin in the gut.

All the factors that led your child to become sick and picky

Recent research has demonstrated that genetics share a complicated relationship with environment in determining our development. We are born with a huge choice of genes, which are covered by special proteins that communicate with our environment, and decide which genes get turned on and off. So, it's our food, water, pollution, thoughts, and other outside factors, that determine our gene expression. This is called epigenetics, meaning "acting upon" genes.

Our food is the most important environmental factor for gene expression, because the nutrients we ingest and absorb, lay the foundation for our most advantageous genetic expression. This starts before we're even born; our mother's diet during pregnancy, and our diet as babies, set up our genetic expressions from the beginning of life. Sadly, toxin exposure before and during pregnancy affects this expression as well.

It may surprise you to learn that a woman's body can release toxins to her child in utero. We used to believe that the amniotic sac was a nearly impenetrable bubble of safety for developing babies. Modern research has shown that the toxins a mother is exposed to during her pregnancy accumulate in her baby too, because they share a blood supply[1]. Babies store toxins from mothers' bodies, and as a result, are born with a toxic load. Some babies are born with a smaller toxic load than others, which gives them stronger health from the beginning.

---

1 http://www.ewg.org/research/body-burden-pollution-newborns/detailed-findings

In most kids, abnormal gut flora was inherited from their mothers and fathers right from birth (nothing to feel guilty about—how were you supposed to know?). Babies are born with an immature immune system, and normal gut flora should be established in roughly the first 20 days of life during the trip through the birth canal and from breastfeeding. Gut flora plays a crucial role in the appropriate development of your baby's immune system.

Most of our immune system is located in the small intestine in lymph tissue called Peyer's Patches, with an army of good gut flora standing guard there. So, if your baby inherited abnormal gut flora or missed out on the trip through the birth canal or breastfeeding, they were immune-compromised from the start. As a result, they likely acquired one infection after another and were prescribed antibiotics each time. Every course of antibiotics killed off some of their gut flora, which further weakened their immune system.

A well-functioning gut makes sure that we're well-nourished and protected from many environmental pitfalls. Healthy gut flora is a big producer of B vitamins, vitamin K2, and other nutrients. When your kid's gut flora is abnormal, he can't digest and absorb food properly and ends up with multiple nutritional deficiencies.

Mineral metabolism is also essential to gut health, but is very complex. In order for the body to absorb minerals, we need gut flora, and in order for the body to use minerals appropriately, we need fat-soluble vitamins. The fat-soluble vitamins A, D, and K are needed for normal growth and development and are also in great demand to deal with toxicity, so there may not be enough to go around. Since we live in a world that's only now slowly overcoming fat phobia, many of us have been limiting fat consumption for our kids from a very young age, which exacerbates this situation.

Most healing diets are rich in natural, minimally-processed fats, which stimulate bile production and excretion into the duodenum (the first segment of the small intestine) at every meal. While it is possible for the gallbladder to return to optimal function for fat digestion, it does take time.

As a result of all these factors—epigenetics, prenatal environment, antibiotics, and nutrient absorption—your kid ended up with very abnormal gut flora and compromised immunity. Abnormal gut flora damages the gastrointestinal tract and causes digestive problems, like colic, diarrhea, constipation, reflux, and bloating. The typical weaning diet that's based on processed grains and processed milk feeds the pathogens in the gut, making the whole situation worse. As the gut wall gets damaged, your child develops allergies and intolerances to foods and other substances. Finally, toxicity originating from the gut invades the brain and other organs in the body.

Toxicity coming from the gut can cause brain dysfunction in children. Most children are born with normal brains, ears, eyes and other sensory organs. Kids use their sensory organs to collect information from the environment and pass it to the brain to be processed. That's how our kids learn to communicate, to behave appropriately, and to fit into the world.

In our compromised kids, their brains are clogged with toxicity, and they're unable to process the information coming from their sensory organs. This information just turns into a "noise," and the child can't make sense of it. Depending on the mixture of toxicity and the severity of the whole problem, a child may become autistic, hyperactive, dyslexic, dyspraxic (unnaturally clumsy), or may develop another mixture of symptoms.

When this toxicity enters other organs in the body, toxins cause physical problems in the child, like eczema, asthma, chronic bladder infections (cystitis) with bed wetting, arthritis, Type 1 diabetes, celiac disease, and others.

Beneficial, transitional, and pathogenic bacteria

Recent research reveals that up to 90 percent of the genetic material and cells in our bodies lives in our gut flora. Essentially, we're just that other 10 percent, a shell providing a habitat for this mass of microbes. In a healthy kid with healthy gut flora, this mass of microbes is dominated by the beneficial or "probiotic" species, which are involved in all kinds of functions in the body.

There are two other kinds of bacteria, though: opportunistic flora, which need to be kept in check by our beneficial flora or they'll cause problems, and transitional flora, which we swallow daily with our food and drink. When our gut is well-protected by beneficial bacteria, this group of microbes goes through your digestive tract without causing harm. But if you're low on beneficial flora, this group of microbes can cause disease. This is what happens when we get food poisoning or traveler's diarrhea.

To give you a hint at what goes wrong when your bacteria gets out of balance, let me tell you what your healthy essential gut flora does for you:

- Protects you from invading transitional flora.

- Maintains the health and integrity of your gut so it doesn't get "leaky."

- Helps you digest your food and absorb nutrients.

- Produces some of your B vitamins and vitamin K.

- Assists detoxification by breaking down toxins and sending them on their way out of your body.

- Modulates your immune system, where they stand as "guards," blocking inappropriate proteins from getting in to your bloodstream.

When your child's gut is dominated by opportunistic or transitional flora, their gut wall starts getting damaged. New gut cells, called enterocytes, aren't born as often as they need to be, and the ones that are born are disabled and can't do their job efficiently. These enterocytes are missing the enzymes that accomplish the last steps in digesting food, which then impairs their digestion and absorption. The structure of your child's gut wall changes and disease can set in, leading to malabsorption, nutritional deficiencies, and food intolerances. Sound familiar?

Pathogens, and the toxins they produce, damage cells in your child's gut and open the spaces between them, which are called the tight junctions. Tight junctions are where enterocytes are tightly "glued" to each other, preventing foods from passing between them. Instead, food is taken inside the enterocytes and analyzed, and then what's useful is let through the other side into the bloodstream.

The tight junctions are formed and maintained by very special proteins, which are like glue. Unfortunately, many pathogenic microbes in abnormal gut flora produce toxins that dissolve the glue and open the tight junctions. The gut then becomes porous and leaky, and substances that shouldn't pass through the gut wall are allowed to get through. Then, your child's immune system finds these partially digested foods in the blood, doesn't recognize them as food, and attacks them. This is how food allergies and intolerances develop.

So, there's nothing wrong with the food; it's the damaged gut lining that causes this phenomenon. Food allergies and intolerances can manifest as many symptoms in the body, from headaches and abnormal behavior to arthritis, and the reaction can show immediately, in a few hours, or in a few days. As these reactions overlap with each other, it becomes impossible for you to figure out what your child's reacting to on any given day.

How diet heals

Now let's look at what happens when you begin focusing on healing and sealing your child's gut lining, and start reversing all this damage.

As the gut flora normalizes, it produces fewer and fewer toxins, so the level of toxicity in your child's body drops. As the gut lining starts healing and sealing, they start digesting food properly before absorbing it, so food allergies and intolerances disappear. Their whole digestive function is restored, so multiple nutritional deficiencies and their symptoms melt away. As they become better nourished, their immune system gets re-balanced, which removes the basis for allergies and autoimmunity in the body; instead of attacking its own tissues, their immune system starts effectively clearing pathogens like candida, viruses, and bacteria out of the body.

Finally, their detoxification system starts working. Everyone is born with a natural detoxification system that cleans our cells, tissues, and organs all the time. In compromised people, this system is broken and doesn't work well, so toxins accumulate.

As your child's detox system starts working again, the levels of various toxins in their body drops, which stimulates more healing and recovery.

The food your child eats makes a difference. Healing diets commonly eliminate inflammatory foods, processed food, and foods that are known sensitivities for the individual, while emphasizing nutrient-dense whole foods, homemade bone broths, and probiotic foods.

Why your child is a picky eater

Kids with poor immunity, autism, sensory processing disorder, asthma, and other ailments are generally picky eaters and mealtime is a nightmare for many parents. Some kids are very fussy and accept only a limited range of foods. Some can't chew properly, and hold food in their mouth for a long time or try to swallow it whole. Some can only suck from a bottle or sippy cup and won't drink from anything else. This is particularly true in the case of autism, but there are a number of reasons a kid might have this problem.

1. *Distorted sensory processing.* If taste buds pass information about food to a brain that's clogged with toxicity, it might taste completely different than expected, and the texture or temperature may not be what was expected.

2. *Cravings for sweet and starchy foods.* These cravings stem from abnormal gut flora, particularly with candida overgrowth. No matter how finicky a child might be, most of them will accept sugary drinks, sweets, breakfast cereals, chocolates, chips, pastas, and white bread. In fact, these are the foods that many kids limit their diet to, and these feed this vicious cycle of abnormal flora and toxicity in their bodies.

3. *The state of the mouth.* Our mouth is home for a large population of microbes that normally protect it from pathogenic bacteria, viruses, and fungi. These good microbes also maintain a healthy state of the mucous membranes and structures in the mouth. Compromised children frequently have abnormal bacterial flora in their mouths, often with an overgrowth of candida and other pathogenic microbes. The activity of this abnormal flora produces a lot of toxins, which are stored in the mucous membranes of the mouth. These alter the function of their taste buds, saliva glands, and other structures. Apart from contributing to the distortion of taste, this process causes a chronic inflammation in the mucous membranes of the mouth, making it a target for the immune system. Due to abnormal mouth flora, these kids frequently have bad breath, red lips and mouth, various sores and ulcers on the cheeks, and a coated tongue. Many foods like raw fruit and veggies, herbs, uncooked nuts and seeds, and cold-pressed oils, have strong detoxifying substances in them, which bind to toxins in the mouth and attempt to remove them. This can create stinging, itching, and burning, as well as unpleasant tastes.

4. *Secretions.* Any secretion from the body, such as saliva, is a way of eliminating toxins. Your child may have a very toxic body, and as some of these toxins get secreted in the saliva, this contributes to toxic load in the mouth, altering the taste and feel of foods.

5. *Challenged muscle structures.* In some cases of autism and other sensory disorders, the inability of the toxic brain to orchestrate normal movements of the muscles in the mouth, tongue, and other structures makes it challenging to chew and swallow. For kids who cannot chew and

swallow properly, foods have to be very soft, and they often vomit. Such severe abnormality is fairly rare, but this problem exists in many sick children. Please have your picky child evaluated by an experienced professional who can determine if your child is struggling with tongue tie, lip tie, or another structural problem that causes them to have a hard time accepting certain foods.

There's no such thing as kid food

Adrienne came to me when she wanted to try getting her kids on the GAPS Intro Diet for the second time. She had attempted once before, and now they were following what she called the Full GAPS Diet. When I had her explain to me in detail exactly what her three children were eating, she described a lot of sweets and what I consider GAPS-friendly junk food.

The biggest problem I saw with her approach was that she was trying to make all of her food "kid friendly." Since her kids only liked things that were sweet, that meant she was adding honey in great quantity to pretty much everything, including the meat stock. In addition, she was spending all kinds of time in the kitchen creating food in "fun" shapes, like dinosaurs, that she thought her girls would more readily accept.

Unfortunately, she wasn't seeing much progress with their sensory issues. She came to see me out of frustration, because for all the work she was putting into these dietary changes, she didn't see great results like she expected.

While the GAPS Diet is a lifestyle change and requires a lot more cooking than most of us are used to, Adrienne was making it even harder on herself by trying to live up to some notion of foods that kids prefer to eat. I'm not saying that food should never be made into creative shapes, but that should not be the norm!

I want to set the record straight about one thing for you: there is no such thing as kid food. Children are human. "Kid foods" are a marketing invention. For 100,000 generations, children ate the same foods as their families after they were weaned from breast milk. Your children need to eat nutritious whole foods, just like you do. Kids are developing and growing like crazy, so they need whole foods more than adults! Children need a steady supply of protein and plenty of fats to fuel the development of their brain as well as the growth of all of their organs, bones, and tissues.

It's perfectly normal for your kids to not like a certain food the first time they try it, but it needs to be offered again and again. It takes somewhere between eight and twelve tries before we decide that we like most things.

If your child has sensory issues, you may need to adjust to their texture or temperature preference at first, but don't fall in to the trap of making everything a "nugget" for the next six years. Keep offering normal foods again and again so they have the opportunity to adjust over time.

Work with a feeding therapist to incorporate strategies for your child's specific sensory issues in conjunction with nourishing foods, so the nutrition and the therapy work together to get better and quicker results.

Let's get real. How many 30-year-olds do you know who still love McDonald's chicken nuggets, fries, or macaroni and cheese, and don't really eat vegetables? I would guess that you probably know lots of adults like this. The sooner you break your kid out of this pattern, the easier it will be for them to accept more food in its natural state, which sets them up for a lifetime of vibrant health.

CHAPTER 2: SHAPE YOUR MINDSET

The most important part of changing your child's diet is your attitude. When you have your mind set to "everything can be figured out," you have no option other than success. That attitude allows you to be creative and flexible, and to trust your intuition.

Healing your child will have its highs and lows. During the lows, it's crucial to keep your eyes on the prize. In order to do that, you'll need to have a clear vision of what future you want for your family. There's no right or wrong vision; this is personal and unique to your dream for your family.

What is your vision for the future?

The very first step on your journey is to decide where your destination is.

To get your imagination percolating, answer these questions about your life as it is right now:

- Are you dealing with behavioral issues daily?

- Do you have a kid on the couch feeling sick more often than not?

- Does one of your kids dominate the family's attention to the detriment of others?

- Is your schedule full of doctor or therapy appointments?

- Are your kids already started on prescription medications?

- Are you afraid to have more children?

- Is it even possible for you to hire a babysitter to get some time for yourself?

- Are your child's opportunities limited if they stay in the developmental state they're currently in?

- What else can't you accept about your kids', or your own, life?

Now envision your life after a healing diet:

- What does your house look like when you wake up in the morning?

- How is your family at the breakfast table?

- Where do your kids go to school?

- How do they interact with friends?

- How are they meeting growth and developmental milestones?

- Are they learning new things easily?

- What activities are *you* focused on during the day?

- Are your evenings peaceful?

- What is your bedtime routine?

- How does everyone in your household function with a full night's sleep?

How far apart are those two scenes?

Don't get discouraged if you're not going to be able to get from here to there overnight. No one does. This is a process that usually takes more than a year. It might be quicker, and you've probably heard stories like that. But it might not. This is your kid. He's unique and special. This is not going to be some cookie-cutter experience.

All you need to ask yourself is, how badly do I want this change, and what's stopping me from having it right now?

Setting goals

Now, let's take that vision and set some measurable goals. "My child is healthy and happy, and eats a wide variety of foods" is a great thing to want, but that doesn't give you something to measure your progress against. If that doesn't happen for two years, what's going to help you stick with this diet in the meantime?

Here are some specific goal examples from my clients:

- Making eye contact.

- No more Epi-Pen use.

- Having a bowel movement every day without enema or a laxative.

- Saying a five-word sentence.

- Conversing.

- Being potty-trained.

- Able to walk barefoot on the grass.

- Eating meat.

- Sleeping in their own bed.

- Playing with other children.

Write down three specific goals on an index card, or in another place, where you can look back and review them from time to time.

Emotional prep

Are you emotionally ready for some ups and downs? The first few days, up to about two weeks, are typically the hardest. Your kid will be emotional, throw tantrums, become lethargic, and otherwise make you feel like the worst parent in the world.

You're not. This will pass. Don't give up.

When your kids grow up, they're going to praise you as the hero who did whatever it took to bring them back to neurotypical opportunities.

The most important thing you can do for your child is stay calm. Set your attitude to, "This isn't personal, it's just something that has to be done. We're following this diet now. Period." Write that on a sticky note that you'll see many times a day, if you need that reminder to keep you strong.

Here's what I want you to prepare for:

1. How will you handle the fits your kids are going to throw? Or, their refusal to eat? Decide your actions in advance. There are suggestions in Chapter 3 to help you decide what will work best for your family and your child.

2. Do you have the support of your family, friends, etc.? Who are they, and how do they support you?

3. Who in your life is negative, thinks this will be torture for your kids, or just doesn't get it? Avoid them for at least the first two weeks. Your life must only include positive and helpful people, who believe in you and agree to help you stay on track. You owe it to your kids to focus on helping them 100 percent right now. Anyone who sees you struggling and encourages you to quit must be shut out of your life briefly. Or forever. You don't ever have to put up with people who bring you down.

4. If your family and friends are curious or receptive, have you given them a copy of your new food list? We can't

expect others to make special food for us, but some people like the challenge and will enjoy creating meals from your recommended foods list.

5. People feel a great sense of satisfaction in helping others. So often people sincerely want to help, but have no idea what to do. Help them help you by creating a list of three things that you always need help with, and keep it ready for when they offer. Examples include: cleaning and chopping a bag of veggies, prepping a simple dish that you can have in the freezer, being a walking buddy, folding towels, or mowing the lawn. The things that seem like drudgery in our own lives are more satisfying to do for others, because they get a thank you and the feeling of being helpful.

6. Send out an email or Facebook post asking for your friends' thoughts, prayers, and positive vibes. Here's an example:

Dear friends,

We're about to begin a special diet with Riley. As you know, he has health challenges. Our family is not willing to accept that this is the best life he can have. We've decided to make a big change, and it's going to be a new way of life. We're excited and nervous, and we don't have time to share all the details right now, but we would love it if you'd keep us in your thoughts and prayers this week as we make the transition.

Thank you,

Brave Family

7. Find one person you can cry with or send a really stressed email to, who can support you calmly (ideally not your spouse since they're going to be in this emotional moment with you). Look to another family member, friend, healthcare practitioner, or an online support group. Make sure they're in on your plans for the new diet in advance, so they're on standby and know what type of emotional support you'll be asking for.

8. If you have a personal or marriage counselor that you see, schedule a session early on, just to check in.

9. Set aside a short time each day to fill yourself back up with motivation and willpower. If you have a regular Tapping, gratitude, meditation, prayer, or exercise practice, keep it going. If you don't, start one now, because self-care is a must.

10. Read a success story every day. Whether you find them on the Internet or in a book about your chosen diet, connecting to other people's success will bring your focus back to the big picture of what's possible.

Prioritizing choices

As much as we want to be perfect, life rarely turns out that way. We can't always do our healing diet perfectly because of finances, time constraints, shared custody, school schedules, etc. How do you know what to prioritize? Your intuition, your budget, and not sweating over every single detail will guide you.

Now, I'm the first person to encourage you to give this healing diet your all, but I also live in reality. Stress is a huge health and joy stealer. *Do your best.*

Top priority is given to your intuition, or your *gut instinct*. This is where following the healing diet yourself for a couple of weeks, before your kids start, comes in handy. It calms your own anxiety and allows you to reconnect with what you know deep down is right. Your intuition will be strongest at the quietest time of day, during meditation, prayer, and walks. Asking the universe for help before you go to sleep at night can lead to you waking up with an "a-ha" the next day.

I typically advise that organic food is the most important part of any diet. If you have a budget shortfall and your intuition tells you that a certain supplement is more important than organic vegetables—go with it. Trust yourself more than you trust me.

If your ex-spouse will only agree to a gluten-free, sugar-free diet during your kids' stay at their house, just go with it. Some healing diet is better than none. Yes, you'll be the strict parent who doesn't allow corn chips, but be the bigger person and keep your rants to yourself. Control what you can and make peace with the rest.

If your kids are on an especially restricted diet and not yet eating fruit (for example) when they get invited to their friends' birthday party, it's a reasonable compromise to make something like a baked apple with cinnamon so your kid doesn't feel totally left out. Just don't confuse the exception with what works on a day-to-day basis. Giving in to your kids' daily or weekly pleas for sweets and treats will only make more work for you in the long run, as it prolongs your child's healing.

Do your best.

Get your kids involved in food prep and cooking

Preparing all your food from scratch takes time. This is a responsibility that should be shared. Set the expectation for your family that everyone eats, and everyone contributes to meals in some way. That can be gardening, shopping, chopping, cooking, setting the table, or cleaning up. No one is exempt, at least not in the long run.

It's probably too much to take on from Day 1 of your new diet, but get your kids involved in cooking. They have to learn this to care for themselves later in life, so start now. Even a toddler can put out napkins. Here are the Montessori recommendations for age-appropriate kitchen tasks[2]. Expect your child to help on their developmental level, and challenge them to do so:

Ages 2-3:

- Throw away trash.

- Set the table.

Ages 4-5:

- Wipe up spills.

- Sort clean silverware.

- Prepare simple snacks.

- Clean kitchen table.

- Dry and put away dishes.

_____

2 http://www.flandersfamily.info/web/age-appropriate-chores-for-children/

Ages 6-7:

- Gather trash and recycling.

- Dust floors.

- Empty dishwasher.

- Peel potatoes or carrots.

- Make salad.

Ages 8-9:

- Load dishwasher.

- Put groceries away.

- Scramble eggs.

- Bake cookies.

- Wipe off the table.

Ages 10-11:

- Clean countertops.

- Deep clean the kitchen.

- Prepare simple meals, such as a soup or pot roast.

Ages 12 and up:

- Mop floors.

- Shop for groceries with a list.

- Cook complete meals.

- Bake bread or cake.

Many food aversions will melt away just by getting your kids involved in a small garden, or taking them to the market and having them pick out foods.

Maybe they like putting the chicken feet in the pot of soup and stirring it like a witch's brew. Running veggies through the juicer or food processor for quick chopping is entertainment for some. Put a kid in charge of checking on the sauerkraut and beet kvass jars and letting the gases escape.

It takes a little bit of effort to teach these things in the beginning. In the long run, they will not only help you, but also provide opportunity for nice conversations as you work together. You'll feel satisfied knowing you've given them life skills they'll always use.

What Dad needs to know about the new diet

Following a healing diet is usually Mom's idea. Mom has been in charge of the decisions in nine out of ten of my clients who've embarked on a healing diet with their kids. That's why I call this section what "Dads need to know about the new diet," but it's really geared towards other people who aren't the initiator and what they need to know about the diet. Dad may not be interested in reading this whole book, so just ask him to read this section as a quick overview that's written just for him.

Here's what Dad needs to know about healing diets:

- They're not a fad. Healing diets are based on the nutrient-dense, whole foods diet that everybody ate before processed foods were invented, coupled with modern research about what types of foods heal the gut and brain and other specific health conditions.

- Your food budget will be bigger. Healing diets emphasize organic and natural foods because they're more nutritious, and processed foods will no longer be eaten. Higher quality food costs more. However, if you've been doing any level of eating out or purchasing prepared meals for quick heating at home, you won't see too much of a difference. In the long run, this will be offset by fewer doctor visits or therapies, and potentially lower schooling costs if your child is in a special education program.

- Things will get worse before they get better. Most symptoms your kids have may get a little bit worse as you begin a new diet. This applies to both physical symptoms like asthma and digestive issues, as well as behavioral issues, sensory issues, and anxiety. We're changing the diet dramatically, and it takes the body a moment to recalibrate. The body also heals in its own way and in its own time, so what might seem like the most pressing issue for you may not be nature's healing priority.

- You have to be 100% on board. This might sound a little woo-woo, but if everyone in the household isn't completely committed to the new diet, I've seen time and time again that families struggle, and kids throw tantrums or exhibit other behavior issues. Our kids know when we're ambivalent or anxious about things. When they sense that both parents are on board and are presenting a united front, the transition to the healing diet goes much, much more smoothly.

- Schedule time for your own self-care or guy-time activities away from distraction. Tapping, gratitude, meditation, prayer, or exercise are good self-care options. Choose an activity that lets you uplift your mind to the big picture goal for your family. Your family needs your resilient "we've got this" attitude, so choose a way to bolster that in yourself.

- Support your partner's need for self-care time. Exercise, alone time, or friend time should be considered a can't-miss appointment for both of you to keep your spirits and energy up.

Don't underestimate the value of your support and commitment to the diet, not only for your kids, but also for your partner. The early adjustment is just that, a big adjustment, and a dramatic change to your lifestyle. Even if you're not in charge of the food preparation, it's important that you educate yourself enough to be comfortable as a cheerleader for your kids while they're following this diet.

CHAPTER 3: CHOOSE YOUR METHOD

How can we address all the different issues that are causing picky eating? By getting your kid nourished, populated with lots of good flora, and detoxified of heavy metals and environmental chemicals. When these three things come together over time, nutritious foods will taste good to her and meal times will be pleasurable.

It's not going to happen right away, and I know you have a lot of anxiety around this issue, or you wouldn't be reading this book. I believe that where there's a will, there's a way, and the fact that you chose to read this book means you have the will.

To get this process started, your child needs your help. On his own, he isn't capable of breaking the vicious cycle of cravings, toxicity, and abnormalities in taste. Once your child has a varied and balanced diet, you can let him refuse a small number of foods he just doesn't like. We all have these likes and dislikes. Just be sure that it's within normal proportions, meaning two to five foods. (I know a lot of... ahem... grown-ups out there who are still very "picky." Those aren't an example of normal.)

There are three methods that I've seen work to get picky kids eating a healing diet, and I'll share each of them with you so you can choose what's best for your family:

1. Applied Behavior Analysis (ABA), a structured method using a reward system.

2. Backing into it by gradually including new foods into their current diet.

3. Cold-turkey Method, or "You're-not-eating-unless-it's-on-the-diet-and-we'll-wait-it-out."

Any of these methods require a lot of determination on your part, but I'm guessing that you have that or you wouldn't be here! Any way you get to a healing diet will bring a huge relief and normality into your family life.

Approximately 80 percent of the parents who come to see me with their children say up front that they can't imagine their child agreeing to eat a special diet. Using these techniques has helped every one of those kids adopt a healing diet in some form. The stress of the first couple of weeks becomes a faded memory, and sitting down to a meal as a family becomes a normal and pleasurable experience, like it's supposed to be.

Applied Behavior Analysis (ABA) method

If you're familiar with Applied Behavior Analysis (ABA), and especially if you're already using it successfully for other things, it's a great option.

ABA is based on common reasoning used by parents for centuries, and you're probably already using the idea with your kids now. When you want your kid to do something, you tell them they get some kind of reward when it's done. Simple examples are:

- Do your homework first, then you can have screen time.

- If you want to go out with your friends on Saturday, you have to do your chores this week.

This isn't bribing, which gives something up front in order to get the outcome you want, but instead reinforces your kids' actions or good behavior with the reward afterward.

When you start using ABA to get your child eating healing foods, he's not going to like it at first. Expect a lot of resistance until he realizes there's no way he's going to "win" the game. If you don't give up in the first difficult days, your child will understand pretty quickly that to get what *he* wants, he has to do something for *you*. As soon as he understands that, your life will be much easier!

Work on introducing one food at a time, since it will be confusing to your child if she is suddenly expected to eat several foods all at once. Choose which food is most important to introduce first, based on your child's nutrition needs. It's smart to start with foods that you think would be easiest for your child to accept. When you've conquered one or two foods and your child's menu starts growing, you'll find that introducing more new foods becomes easier and easier. Soon, your child will be eating a varied and nourishing diet!

Don't get frustrated by the initial resistance you'll get from your kid. The first week or two will seem like an eternity in the moment, but when you look back, it will seem like it all happened in the blink of an eye. Remember that thousands of parents have implemented ABA programs with their children and survived the initial stage of tantrums! Nobody can teach a child who doesn't comply with anything you ask her to do. Once you've won the first battle, you've opened your child up to accepting change and this new way of doing things, which means that you now have a child you can teach.

Now, let's talk about how we can apply this method to introduce new foods to different types of children.

ABA with a child who is non-verbal or has severe language problems

In the beginning, use your child's favorite foods as rewards for eating the new food. The reward food examples listed, like chocolate and crackers, are foods that may not be part of the healing diet, but in the initial stages when you're teaching your child the whole ABA concept, you can use whatever works.

If you can get your child to eat the new foods without using food as a reward, do so! If they respond to things like stickers, toys, videos, or play time, that's even better. Once they understand the rules of the game, you want to move to rewards that are allowed on the healing diet.

Food reward example:

1. Show your child the food or reward that she likes the most—a piece of chocolate, crackers, cereal, or macaroni and cheese. Put it out of her reach, but keep it in clear view.

2. Offer her one bite of the new food that you want her to try. Stay completely calm while you ignore tantrums, screaming, or crying. Don't give her what she wants until she's had one bite of the food, and don't let her leave the table. Don't be angry about the resistance you get. It's your job to offer the food and embody the fact that these are the new rules of life, and you're just calmly enforcing them.

3. When she's had one mouthful of the new food, or even just tasted it, give her the reward with lavish praise! Offer affection, cheering, or whatever your child would appreciate hearing most from you. Then, let her leave the table.

4. After a short break of a few minutes, repeat this process again. Just work on one mouthful at a time, reward her, and let her go.

5. In a few minutes, repeat this again.

Give your child just a small amount of the reward food, like one or two fish crackers, a small bite of chocolate, etc. If she comes back for more, get her to eat another bite of the new food before rewarding her with another one of her treat foods. And remember to only work on one new food at a time.

Her preferred foods are now available *only as rewards for eating the healing foods*. If you give them to your kid at other times, she'll wait for the time when she can get them without any effort or compromise on her part.

After your child starts taking one bite of the new food you've been working on without any protest, the next step will be requiring two bites of the same food for one reward. You may spend a few days, a week, or even more on the "one bite" stage. Every child takes a different amount of time. After you've conquered two bites, move to three bites for the same reward, and so on, slowly increasing the number of bites until she eats the whole meal.

If your child can be motivated by any dessert ideas allowed on your healing diet in the beginning, then great! Forget about the food examples I gave and start there. Besides favorite foods, you can use anything else your child likes as a reward for getting them to the new food.

Video reward example:

1. If your child likes to watch a particular video, put the video on for five minutes and then pause it.

2. Offer him the bite of new food you want to introduce into his diet. Don't switch the video back on again until he's eaten the bite. Don't give in to tantrums, screaming, or crying, When your child has eaten the bite, give him lavish and enthusiastic praise.

3. Switch the video back on for a few minutes. After a few minutes, repeat the procedure again.

If your child isn't particularly interested in videos, use whatever toys, books, stickers, or games that do interest them.

In general, obsessive play and self-stimulation—like spinning or pacing—that are used as a way to soothe stress,   shouldn't be encouraged in children with autism. However, if that is the *only thing* that would motivate your child, you can use them as a reward for eating new foods in the beginning.

ABA for a child without language challenges

With children who don't have communication challenges, the ABA method is similar but much easier to implement, because you have more tools available to reason with him. You can explain that he has to eat the new food first in order to get what he wants (e.g., preferred foods, screen time, a game, or a toy).

I don't use non-allowed foods like chocolates or crackers as rewards with these kids. You can use homemade desserts or fruits from the new diet, and tell your child, like your mom probably said to you as a kid, "Finish your dinner so you can have dessert." Even better than food rewards are using more sophisticated rewards like games, toys, or special outings.

Just like non-verbal children, it's important to start with small, achievable targets like one bite or a small piece of food. If you try to start with a full plate of food that your child hates, you're going to fail because the reward requires too much work. Once your child accepts a small amount of food for a reward, move to larger and larger portions.

Be patient and consistent! *Do not give in* to whining, complaining, or tantrums! If she doesn't eat the new food, she doesn't get the reward. It's as simple as that. You have to be firm and kind. I cannot overstate this.

Choose the food and size of the bite carefully, because once you've asked your child to eat the one bite of food, you can't back off or allow any negotiation or manipulation. If your kid "wins" one food battle, you have not only lost the food war, but you've set a precedent that they can use the same tactic to win on other issues, and their resistance will grow stronger. If you give in and then try to start up again later, you will have double or even triple the resistance. Start strong so you only have to go through this process once. If your child refuses one bite of new food and doesn't seem to care that he or she didn't get the reward, it means you've chosen the wrong reward. Choose a reward that your child cares about enough to do *anything* to get it.

No matter how motivating the reward, never forget to add your lavish and enthusiastic praise and hugs! Your child has to feel that she's done something *really good* when she had that mouthful of the new food, so let her see how happy and proud she's made you by eating the healing food. Your enthusiasm, combined with the reward given at the same time, will make this experience something for her to look forward to, and to anticipate with pleasure at the next meal time.

Keep in mind that most of the time kids have to taste a food several times before they can truly decide if they like it. As his gut flora begins to normalize, a normal sense of taste returns, most cravings go away, and he will start liking new and different foods. If you work on a food that he accepts easily, jump for joy!

It's important to keep this whole process positive and filled with curiosity. Talk to your child and explain why you want them to eat these foods, and how it will help their bodies and their moods. Older children and teenagers are often very aware and self-conscious of their moods and truly want to be "normal." You can talk about this at every meal, using language and phrases on your child's level. Ask them questions about how they feel after eating, to get them connecting with how food makes them feel.

- Do they feel creative?

- Are they happy or grumpy?

- Are they forgetful?

- Do they feel clumsy?

- Does their tummy hurt?

- Do they have energy, or do they feel like lying on the couch?

If you're already doing an ABA program with your child at home or at school, use ABA to start your child on your new diet. Make feeding an area for your therapist to work on in the sessions. All you have to do is cook the food and bring it to therapy.

Backing into the new diet

If your child, teenager, or adult child with autism may become aggressive and harm you, themselves, or things around the house, use the method of backing into the new diet. If your picky kid is a teenager, this may be the only method they'll agree to.

The pros of backing into the healing diet are that it can be easier for your child to adapt to *and* easier for you to commit to. You're not overhauling your whole life at once, just taking one step at a time to get to a new eating lifestyle.

The con of backing into the healing diet is that it can take a long time to get there, depending on where you're starting from. There's nothing that says you can't use this method for a while and then switch to ABA or Cold Turkey if you feel ready for one of those methods later.

Backing into a healing diet doesn't have a set of specific steps, because it all depends on what you want to trial and what you think your child might tolerate a little bit of, then increasing the number and amount of healing foods over time.

You're starting from your child's diet the way it is today and slowly incorporate healing foods, while crowding out non-healing foods over time. Simple examples are, adding in soup once a week, making sausage for breakfast instead of oatmeal, or switching out wheat-based muffins for nut-flour based muffins.

Guidelines for how to transition to a healing diet with your child by backing into it:

1. Choose any new food that you'd like to *add* to their diet or think you can sneak into something they already eat.

2. Slowly work in new foods regularly, possibly starting with healing diet sweets and treats or bread while "running out" of their normal treats.

3. If they like fruit, encourage more fruit over cookies and candy.

4. Sneak in healing foods and supplements any way you can. For example, adding five drops of broth in a fruit smoothie

or blending a chunk of avocado into their ketchup *is* a start.

5. Consider an ABA reward-system if it will work for a specific new food that you can't sneak in, or that they won't agree to eat readily.

6. Be comfortable with small, progressive steps.

7. When you've seen some progress, and you and your child are both in a stable emotional place to push it a little, insist that she tries something new.

8. Strongly limit eating out.

9. Try denying them a preferred food or restaurant until a certain date on the calendar and increase the time in between. Some kids are okay as long as they know they can have their preferred food again on a specific date that they can look forward to.

This method may take one to two years of transitioning before you get to a point where you are completely on the healing diet. That's still progress. If the alternative is never doing it, what do you have to lose?

The Cold Turkey method or "You're-not-eating-unless-it's-the-new-diet-and-we'll-wait-it-out"

One of the drawbacks of ABA and backing into it is that it can take a looong time. It all depends on the child and how quickly they'll accept new foods, or how long and consistently you're willing to work on the ABA process. For working parents who don't have an ABA therapist to work with them, it can be almost impossible. There are also parents who've tried ABA in other areas and found that it really didn't work for them, and don't want to use it for their new diet.

The alternative I offer is the Cold Turkey method, which consists of only offering healing foods to your child. Period.

This is my favorite method because it's the quickest way to get picky kids on a healing diet, especially younger kids on the autism spectrum or with sensory processing disorder.

The difficulty with this method is that it's always accompanied by three to ten days of almost no food consumption. There's a battle of wills and *you* must win. The strategy is that children will not starve themselves to death. We keep them hydrated, continually offer healing food options, and at some point, they'll realize that you are absolutely serious about this and they'll try the new foods. In a week or so, they will be eating a healing diet. It probably won't look like the perfect, step-by-step version of your chosen diet, but they will be eating only foods allowed on that diet.

This method is just as hard as ABA—and more intense. Your child will throw a tantrum, they'll complain that they're starving, they'll threaten you, and eventually they'll wear themselves out and lie on the couch. They'll be extremely fatigued and zombie-like. They won't play or show interest in their normal activities.

You will feel like the cruelest parent on Earth (it's totally not true!), which is why *everyone* in your household (and at school) must agree 100 percent with the Cold Turkey method before you start. If your child thinks they can get someone else to take pity on them and sneak them their preferred food, they will be extra resistant to the new foods.

It is critical that you remain calm and non-judgmental in front of your kid at all times. Do not yell or fight with your kid to get him to eat. Your body language should communicate that you didn't make these rules; it's just your job to uphold them.

Cold Turkey method steps:

1. Choose a start date and make sure it's during a week when you don't have to work or have any other commitments. Getting your child on this new diet is your only job this week.

2. Remove *all* non-diet foods from your home, but particularly from anywhere your child will see them. If Dad and siblings aren't going to follow the new diet, they must eat their bagels, chips, cookies, and pasta elsewhere.

3. Have a selection of the new diet's most crucial savory foods on hand.

4. Offer your child one of these foods. They'll probably refuse it. When they ask for food later, offer them the same thing.

5. While they are fasting (refusing to eat), make sure that they stay hydrated by drinking water with a pinch of natural sea salt in it. If they won't drink water, offer herbal tea. If that doesn't work, offer them something like watered-down, fresh-pressed carrot and celery juice. Still no luck? Make some lemonade with fresh-pressed lemon juice, water, a pinch of natural sea salt, and a little dab of honey. They can drink as much as they want of any of these.

6. Do not offer fruit, nuts, or any baked goods. Savory foods and juice only.

7. Eat the new foods in front of them without making a big deal out of it, and don't require them to be at the table.

8. Repeat this each day and do not give up. If your child accepts food on day three or earlier, you've had an exceptionally easy time—congrats! Five to seven days is the norm.

You may take a little leeway in getting your child to eat the new foods, if your diet allows that. For example, if your diet requires soup, you may "disassemble" the soup and offer them the cooked meat and veggies on a plate with broth in a cup.

If your child has texture sensitivities, make a recipe that you think will suit them and offer that. Some kids will first accept food in the form of a smoothie and some only in the form of a meatball. Some will drink juice and some gag on it.

It's important for you to figure out what texture and temperature of food works for your child. Keep in mind that any type of food or recipe can be made in other forms. There's no reason that you can't purée your cooked hamburger and make it into some kind of shake or soup consistency. If soup is a key part of the diet you've chosen and your child won't drink things of a soup consistency, then you'll cook all of your meat and vegetables in meat stock, so that they're at least getting some stock dripping from all the foods that they eat. Check out Chapter 12 for specific ideas for your challenge.

There are two directions this method most often goes depending on the kid: "everything in a smoothie" or "only meat." Either is fine for a while. If they accept a smoothie, put a bit of everything else in it. For example, you can sneak supplements, broth, and fermented foods in it. If they'll only eat meat or meatballs, add in pureed or minced veggies, supplements, 10 percent pureed or ground organ meat, and cook them in broth.

No matter what method you are using, when your child eats a few bites of something, use that as a springboard for adding more foods. For example:

- If he'll eat a meatball or hamburger, cook them all in stock and add minced or pureed veggies and organ meats to the mixture.

- If she likes a juice smoothie texture, then you can sneak other types of foods into that, like a spoonful of unseasoned chicken stock or a teaspoon of sauerkraut.

Is this the same as consuming a therapeutic amount of the necessary food? No, but it's a starting point, and you'll rejoice in small victories. Some healing food is better than none.

Keep offering other food options daily. Maybe use a little ABA method with the smoothie as a reward. Let them see you continue to eat other healing foods in front of them. Some kids will ask to try something their parents are eating only when their parents stop offering it.

Celebrate all the foods they eat, and keep expanding on variety and texture every week. It may take several weeks of simple foods before your kid builds up enough nutrition, and begins detoxifying to the point that he can tolerate new textures.

Choose the method here that you think will work best for your child *and* for you. They each have their difficulties, so make sure you're emotionally prepared to stick with whichever choice you make. If you give up and decide to start again, you'll face two to three times the original resistance, so make sure you've set yourself up to succeed by preparing in advance and knowing what to expect as you begin.

CHAPTER 4:
GET PREPARED

When you have a kid that's unwell partly due to diet and lifestyle, you are most likely suffering some of the same ill effects. But like all parents, you want them to get well more than you want that for yourself. You want to see them living the happy eczema-food-allergy-immune-challenge-autism-FREE life that every kid deserves. That's why you're thinking about a healing diet.

Well, I'm going to ask you to hold on a second. One of the best tips I have for parents who want to start a gut healing diet for themselves and their kids, is to begin the diet yourself first. Again and again and again, I have seen parents put their children on a healing diet while not following it themselves, and the parents are so filled with anxiety and indecision, that their child's progress is seriously hindered.

You know how on an airplane you're supposed to put on your air mask before you help your child? You starting this diet before them is just like that. You'll be better able to help your kids if you help yourself first.

There are three reasons why this will make for a wildly successful experience for your family:

1. You'll get through your initial crummy-feeling-time while everyone else is still "normal." You're probably already aware that the first three days to two weeks of a healing diet is a time that people don't feel so hot. I call it a healing reaction, but sometimes it's referred to as die-off or detox symptoms. Whatever you want to call it, you're likely to feel under the weather, fatigued, and some combination of hungry and angry that I call "hangry." It would be extra-stressful to have your whole family feeling like that at the same time and complaining to you, the evil person who's torturing them by denying them their universal right to eat potato chips.

2. You'll get the hang of the cooking and feel more confident about it. As a grown-up, you're more forgiving if the cooking takes longer than expected or if things don't taste just as you planned. With your kids, you might have a hard time getting them excited about the food, so you want it to be as good as it can from the beginning. If you follow the new eating plan for a while before you start with your kids, you'll feel more confident about your repertoire of new food options, and that will reduce your meal time stress.

3. Your energy will be better before you have to deal with your kids' crummy-feeling-time. Now that you've made

it through those first couple of weeks, your thinking is clear, your digestive system feels better, and your energy is sustained. This gives you the stamina to wade through the tough times as you begin your kids on this new eating plan. Now, it's their turn to feel under the weather, fatigued, and hangry. You'll have both the energy and the experience to see them through this tough time and the understanding of what wonderful things lay on the other side for them.

When I suggest that you start your healing diet before your kids, I don't mean you need to be completely healed before they begin. Instead, I'm suggesting that you follow the new diet for two to three weeks before you start the rest of your family on it. I can give you countless stories of how well this works, but I'll share one of my favorites with you.

Ellie is the mother of Jason, a two-and-a-half-year-old boy with an autism pre-diagnosis. Ellie knew that she needed the GAPS Diet because she had some digestive problems and had learned enough about GAPS to know that it runs in the family. Ellie was also nursing Jason, so she knew that she couldn't start with the GAPS Intro Diet but needed to do the Full GAPS Diet for some relief.

She began the Full GAPS Diet and followed it on her own for almost three months before she started Jason on the Intro Diet. In those three months, Ellie had incredible gains in her digestive function; more importantly, her energy level skyrocketed.

When she first thought about doing GAPS, she was overwhelmed by the question, "How am I going to make all this food and keep up with all these new activities on the GAPS Diet, in addition to working and going to school?" After she began and regained tons of energy, it was a snap to do all those things. By the time Jason started the Intro Diet, she had the recipes down and knew how to structure her daily routine in a way that made GAPS easy to stick with.

When we started Jason on the GAPS Intro Diet, he refused food for almost a week, which was extremely stressful. Because Ellie had gone through the diet, had seen the benefits herself, and knew how hard it was for her in the beginning, she was able to work through her fear and guilt and stick with it for Jason.

He lost his autism diagnosis in less than one year.

Practical matters

Plan for your kids' school lunches. Are their teachers aware of the new dietary restrictions and are they on board with them? They can't police every child's food, but they can be helpful in making sure your kid isn't swiping gluten-filled snacks from friends. Unfortunately, sugary treats are a frequent occurrence at most schools. It will take a lot of parents working with the school systems to turn toward treat activities rather than treat foods.

For now, talk to your kids' teachers to find out what alternative treats you can leave with them for your kids. Be willing to compromise here if required. For example, make a fruit-based treat even if that's not what you're eating at home. If it's a real struggle, it's better to provide something so your kids don't feel too left out of cupcake time. An imperfect healing diet is better than none.

Costs. Preparing to start a healing diet can require a bit of coin up front, but it's an excellent investment in your future health and well-being. You can be successful at any budget level. (If you feel stuck on this step, go back and review Chapter 2 again.)

1. What is your monthly food budget? Whole foods can be cheaper than restaurant and packaged meals, but you will "pay" more in preparation time.

2. When you have to make choices based on your budget, keep in mind:

   a. *What type of food is it and how contaminated might it be?* For example, I would never eat organ meats from animals raised in confinement and given feed with hormones and antibiotics. Onions, however, test as having less pesticide residue than other veggies, so I may not always buy them organic.

   b. *How often do you eat it and what is the cost per serving?* If I pay $6 a dozen for pasture-raised eggs, and two eggs is a serving, that's $1. If I buy a steak for $9 and split it with my husband, that's $4.50 a serving. Eggs are a staple for us, and steak is a treat.

   c. *How much nutrition do you get for the cost?* Organic apples are a good source of Vitamin C and fiber. A serving is usually one whole apple, which may cost $2 if it's large. Red cabbage has Vitamin C, Vitamin K, B Vitamins, and small amounts of several minerals. You can enhance this further by turning a $2 head of cabbage into 2 quarts of sauerkraut. While apples are perfectly healthy, they aren't as densely packed with nutrients. Red cabbage is the better buy.

3. Do you need to buy any new kitchen equipment? Do that as soon as possible, because the time savings of an efficient kitchen are well worth it.

4. How often will you need to buy supplements or other special supplies? Make these part of your budget, too.

Timing

There's never a "perfect" time, but some really are better than others.

1. Do you have a vacation, school assignment, work project, family coming to visit, or anything else that really needs your time and attention instead? Do your kids have a special activity, project, performance, etc., within the next few weeks? These would not be an ideal time to start your new diet.

2. Is it summer? Summer may be the only time of year you can control what your kids eat all day, so it can be an optimal start time.

3. Is there a school break coming up? Starting your new diet when your kids have at least a week off a school is the best option.

Prioritize sleep and rest. Our body uses these downtimes to repair and regenerate. Going to bed 15 minutes earlier or planning a nap each day can add up to better health and stress management for your kid and yourself. What can you put on the back burner in order to take time for yourself? What's the right mix of extracurricular activities for the kids during this time? They'll need some exercise and play, preferably outdoors, but obligations every evening may be too strenuous. They'll need to reserve some energy for healing.

Community resources

Allow yourself an hour to seek out these community resources and write down what you find out so you can refer to it later.

Find at least one restaurant in town that serves something acceptable on your new diet (I promise you'll need this in a pinch!). Look for a place with high-quality, local or organic food. You may find options by using gluten-free, organic, or Paleo in the search, for example. You may not find a perfect restaurant, but you won't fall for pizza or pasta in a panic. It's also nice to give your cook a night off here and there and eat with others.

Kitchen prep

It took me about three years to upgrade all my cheap cookware and plastic containers. Since then, cooking has been much easier, more enjoyable, and less stressful! My best advice is to research and purchase the best kitchen equipment that you can. For years, I owned only one knife, but it was an excellent quality Cutco knife. This served me better than a whole set of cheap knives. I always look for materials that are safe, clean easily, and will last a long time. The time and effort you will save on cleaning and replacing broken things is worth the money!

Things to check and buy, if needed:

- Cookware and kitchen equipment.

- Water filter or other source of purified water.

- Lunch containers and thermoses.

- Freezer space. The more the better! You can take advantage of better prices on grass-fed meat, and you can make more meals in advance.

Get in the habit of cleaning dishes as you go. Letting things pile up in the sink leads to feeling overwhelmed. And do some research on how to reheat food without a microwave, since food is tastier when warmed on the stove or in the oven. Plus, you don't end up with hot spots that can burn your child's mouth (see *Resources*).

Cooking and food prep skills

Search for cooking classes online or locally. Have an enthusiastic cook in your family or circle of friends? Ask them for a tutorial. Most people who love cooking love to share their passion with others! Getting some tips on how to chop veggies quickly or making sauerkraut with a pro is super-helpful.

Take a few weeks in advance to try out the foods you need to make for the new diet. That way, if you make a mistake, you have time to try again. When it comes to cultured and fermented foods, it's very common to mess them up on the first try, so start with a small batch. They're part science and part art. Practice makes perfect.

Not planning to start your new diet for a couple of months or more? Choose one new recipe a week to try. You'll build up a great repertoire of recipes and get your family used to new things.

Go through your fridge and cupboards and toss out the non-allowed foods. Make sure to check the labels for sugar and other unsuspected additives. A couple of hours spent on this will free up space for your new habits to take root, and will cut down on the possibility of giving into desperate cravings for off-limits foods in the beginning.

Supplement prep and other supplies

Do you have the supplements you need? Will you need special detox items? An enema kit? Non-toxic shampoo and body soap?

Tips and customizations for picky kids

- Choose a start date when one parent, or ideally both parents, can take a week off work and all evening obligations. Make this a week when your kids are off school, too.

- Everyone in your household needs to be on board with the new diet for this child. If Dad, mother-in-law, or anyone else thinks that you are torturing your child, considers you crazy, or has other negative things to say, this is going to be extremely challenging, and there's a good chance that you will not stick with it. The first week of a healing diet with kids who are picky is extremely stressful, and people will attempt to talk you out of it if they don't understand how it works and what the vision is for your future. Do whatever it takes to get them on board, and don't start until they are.

- Add in some of the new foods for your kids to try before you embark on the diet. This gives your kids a chance to taste a few things without the pressure of having it be the only thing they eat. They'll have some familiarity with it before you remove their processed carbohydrates.

- Plan for three to ten days of your child not eating any food. I am not kidding. This is extremely common. I promise, your child will not starve.

- Do not give up! If you give into non-allowed foods, your kid knows they "won" this round, and if you re-try later, you can expect twice as long without food. This is not a guess, but what I have seen time and time again in my practice!

If you're anxious to get started on some healing foods now, add a few new foods or recipes into your plan for this week. You'll get some of the healing or nourishing benefits now, and give your kids a head start on the eight to twelve tries it takes before they'll know if they like a new food.

Are you ready to make this new diet your second full-time job for a while? Every new job is overwhelming for the first month or two, because you have so much to learn and manage. Expect it to take that long before you feel like you have everything handled and your household becomes a smooth-running machine. Read on for what to expect in these early weeks.

CHAPTER 5: WHAT TO EXPECT AS YOU BEGIN

It's typical for kids on the autism spectrum or with other sensory processing disorders to eat only a few foods, most of which are simple carbohydrates and maybe one type of processed meat, often from specific brands. So, it makes sense that your biggest reservation about starting a gut healing diet is that it will be impossible to get them to eat the new foods. This is a normal fear, and in my experience, picky kids always resist new foods at first.

What to expect during the first week of a new diet with picky kids

In my Nutritional Therapy practice, I most often use the Cold Turkey Method, which is the most intense method. I'd like to share what to do and what you can expect in the first week or two.

We start with the most crucial healing foods, but many kids won't eat the soup or might even gag when we try to feed it to them. You can work around that.

- Leave out known food allergies and sensitivities for the first three months. After three months of healing, you can trial the sensitive foods one at a time and see if they are tolerated.

- Your picky eater will refuse food or eat very minimally for three to ten days. Children will generally fast, or "cleanse," in the beginning if they can't eat the foods they're addicted to. If your kid puts any bite of food in their mouth and actually swallows it within three days, consider yourself the luckiest parent in the world! In most cases, it takes five to seven days before super-picky kids will start eating any of the healing foods.

- The most important thing to do during this first week is keep your kid hydrated.

  » Filtered water with a little pinch of salt added for electrolyte balance is ideal.

  » If they won't drink water, you can offer homemade lemonade with fresh lemon juice, filtered water, sea salt, and a little touch of honey.

  » Not a fan of that? Try fresh pressed vegetable juices, maybe with a little bit of green apple added for sweetness.

- You and the rest of the family should eat the new foods in front of them without pressuring them to eat. I've worked with kids who will show interest in these foods when the parents are eating them and not offering it to them.

- Eliminate sweets and treats unless you're using them for ABA or using honey for low blood sugar (see Chapter 10).

- When your child starts eating some kind of food, let them have as much as of it as they want at first. You'll work in more variety later on.

- Reference Chapter 10 for Troubleshooting Issues and Chapter 12 for My Child Won't... for any issues that come up. There will be issues, but they vary with the child.

The most important thing—*don't give up!*

Have a conversation with all the adults in your household to make sure everyone is still 100 percent on board with the new diet. If your kid senses any arguments or doubt or that someone might "take pity on them" and give in to their cravings, they'll hold out for that. Everyone's energy must be completely "in" for this change.

Go with their texture and temperature preferences in the beginning. The more we can sneak in to begin with, the more nutrients they're going to be taking in an absorbing, and the easier it is for them to detoxify and to have their pickiness melt away over time.

Be aware that this isn't simple, and it isn't a straight line to eating all kinds of foods willingly. Keep experimenting, and you'll find ways to get your kids to agree to try a bite of something new now and then.

Even for neurotypical kids without sensory issues, it's common for them to need to try a food seven to eight times before deciding that they like it. With kids who have sensory issues, we can expect this number to be something like 20 to 30 times or more.

You are not the worst parent in the world

On the first week of the new diet with your picky eaters, you're going to feel like a horrible parent who's torturing your kids. This is temporary, and it's completely untrue. You are doing this for their long-term health and happiness, and while this might be the longest week of your life right now, when you look back a few months down the road and see the progress that your child has made, it will be worth every moment of stress, uncertainty, and pain.

Keep your eye on the big picture of that vision you have for your family. Your child is on her way to regaining her health and functioning at her highest possible level!

Here are the negatives to expect that first week:

- *Feeling under the weather.* This is the most common thing parents report. When your child begins a healing diet, you might think they're coming down with a cold or flu. They might be feverish, achy, have a bit of a sore throat, or feel generally yucky. This "under the weather" feeling might last anywhere from three to ten days.

- *Constipation.* It might not set in during the first few days, but don't be surprised when it does. Your child is likely eating less food and possibly less fiber then they're used to, and their body has lost all the 'crutches' that may have allowed them to go to bathroom easily before (maybe too easily?).

- *Feeling and acting emotionally.* Early on in the diet, your child will be hangry. They'll be hungry for everything they can't eat and angry because you only offer them what's

66

allowed on the healing diet. Breaking a sugar addiction is like breaking a drug habit. It's ugly, and those microbes that are being starved are pissed. There will be tantrums and crying. Expect that this is just part of the process and it will pass. Warn everyone in your household about this in advance. If other people in your home aren't following the diet, your child will be jealous and resentful toward them and will steal their food.

- *Nausea and Vomiting.* These don't happen to everybody, but don't be surprised if they happen to your child. They can be due to a drop in blood sugar or the inability to digest fats well. You'll find detailed information on these troubleshooting issues in Chapter 10.

- *Fatigue.* Your child being completely lethargic or zombie-like is absolutely normal. Every single parent says to me, "This isn't like my kid. They never act like this." Every child on the beginning of a healing diet goes through this. All the energy they have is turned inward toward healing, just like when they have the flu. It's temporary.

Here are the positives to expect that first week:

- *Stomach pain disappears.* You've removed pretty much everything that causes food reactions, and you're adding in healing agents. This all adds up to a beautifully-feeling belly in the early stages of the new diet.

- *Diarrhea improves.* For most people, this disappears during the first week. If your new diet is low fiber or eliminates grains, that source of irritation is gone. If your child is still having diarrhea within a few days, see Chapter 10 for ideas.

- *Sleep is better.* For some kids, this is simply due to the removal of sugar from the diet. For others, it's the addition of nutrient and mineral-dense foods. This happens very quickly in children, especially for those who are on the autism spectrum.

Hopefully, you've gained a little peace of mind by knowing what you have to look forward to. I don't want to scare anyone about the first week of a new diet, but I do want you to make a realistic plan for what you'll need to deal with, and to also realize that it will be temporary and you *will* get through any difficulties. The vibrant, healthy child who's awaiting you on the other side of this is absolutely worth it, so keep your eyes on the prize!

CHAPTER 6: ANTICIPATE REACTIONS

It can sometimes be difficult to distinguish what type of reaction your child is having when they begin a new diet. Is it low blood sugar, die-off, detox, food sensitivity, or just a temporary digestive reaction? What are common reactions to new diets?

Blood sugar issues

Low blood sugar, or hypoglycemia, can be an issue at the start of a healing diet. Most sick kids are sugar or carbohydrate addicts. If your child eats mostly carbohydrates with very little meat or fat, you should prepare for low blood sugar episodes. Your child's metabolism has been running strictly on the rollercoaster of frequent carb intake, and eliminating those will be a shock to their system.

Think of our energy production system, or metabolism, like building a fire. Carbohydrates and sugar are like kindling. If you want to keep a fire going with only kindling, you have to toss more on the fire very frequently. Fat is like putting a log on the fire that will burn for hours. When your metabolism runs off of fat, you don't have to add more to or "tend" the fire very often.

Fat is the preferred fuel of our bodies, but when we're switching over to it, there can be some sputtering as it relearns how to use it and digest it.

Our aim on a balanced diet is for your child to have a flexible fat-burning metabolism, but it takes some time to switch over to that naturally and efficiently. In the early days, you must keep an eye out for signs of low blood sugar.

Signs of low blood sugar

If you see any of the following symptoms in your child, intervene with one of the recipes below:

- Shakiness.

- Nervousness or anxiety.

- Sweating, chills, and clamminess.

- Irritability or impatience.

- Confusion, including delirium.

- Rapid/fast heartbeat.

- Lightheadedness or dizziness.

- Hunger and nausea.

- Sleepiness.

- Blurred/impaired vision.

- Tingling or numbness in the lips or tongue.

- Headaches.

- Weakness or fatigue.

- Anger, stubbornness, or sadness.

- Lack of coordination.

- Nightmares or crying out during sleep.

- Seizures.

- Unconsciousness[3].

Low blood sugar can be dangerous, so stay on top of this.

Managing low blood sugar

Have one of the suggestions below on hand, or plan to feed your child a small amount of food very frequently, until they work through this.

It's ideal to include a simple carbohydrate, like honey, with a fat that doesn't require much to digest, like coconut oil or ghee, so you get both the kindling and the log together.

---

3 http://www.diabetes.org/living-with-diabetes/treatment-and-care/blood-glucose-control/hypoglycemia-low-blood.html

Coconut Oil-Honey Mixture: Thoroughly mix 1 cup of softened unrefined coconut oil with 2 tablespoons of raw honey. Store this in a glass jar and offer your child a spoonful every 20 minutes, or as needed, to keep them from displaying the above symptoms. You can use ghee if they are sensitive to coconut oil.

Apple or Carrot Juice: Use a juicer to make fresh apple or carrot juice and offer them half a cup of juice at the first sign of low blood sugar. It's ideal to include a spoon of fat, like coconut oil or ghee, along with this. If you're out somewhere, you can use an organic, store-bought juice.

People usually think that they'll be addicted to the coconut-oil honey mixture because it tastes yummy. Since your child is eating nourishing foods in addition to this, and their metabolism is adjusting, you'll find that this remedy is quickly forgotten. These interventions are typically needed for one to two weeks.

Die-off reactions

Fermented foods and therapeutic strength probiotics may produce a so-called "die-off" reaction. As the probiotic bacteria make it to the digestive system, they start destroying pathogenic bacteria, viruses, and fungi. When these pathogens die, they release toxins that cause your child's symptoms, so whatever is typical for them may temporarily get worse until it clears from their system. Symptoms might include increased self-stimulating behavior, skin issues, diarrhea, or fatigue. Die-off reactions typically occur 20 minutes to two hours after ingesting fermented foods or probiotic supplements, especially if it's a new type or larger quantity.

How to calm a die-off reaction

If your child is overwhelmed by a die-off reaction, a capsule of activated charcoal can be taken in food or a drink to bind the toxins. Activated charcoal is a blood purifier often used for first aid. When you take it in response to a die-off reaction, it binds to the toxins that have been released and are circulating in the blood. It holds on to them until they can be safely released through the bowel (you may notice black streaks in your child's stool).

A word of caution when taking activated charcoal: you don't want to have your child take this all the time to try and prevent feeling a die-off reaction, because in addition to binding to toxic metals, it also binds to necessary minerals. This isn't a problem if you only take activated charcoal when you need it, because it tends to be just a dozen times or so.

If activated charcoal doesn't seem to help, try modified citrus pectin instead. It's also a binder, and doesn't chelate (bind to) needed minerals, but it is more costly. Pectin is a naturally-occurring, soluble dietary fiber found in most plants. These long-branched polysaccharides have been modified into shorter lengths of soluble fiber that dissolve easily in water, and are readily absorbed into the bloodstream. These show promise in binding to heavy metals, allowing for urinary excretion.

You can also have your child take a detox bath. Some toxicity will leave her body through her pores and go into the bath water, while at the same time, she'll take in some nutrients from whatever you've added to the bath. That takes some burden off her liver and kidneys, which detoxify the substances that were released. (See Chapter 10 for specific bath additive suggestions.)

Wait until the reaction has passed completely before trying the fermented food or probiotic capsule again. On the next attempt, cut the amount of fermented food and/or capsule of probiotic down by 50 percent and see if the reaction happens again. If it does, repeat the process, cutting down by 50 percent again. If there's no reaction, build up from that level very slowly. It's fine to start with just a few drops of fermented food or a pinch of probiotic powder. In the beginning, one of my clients could only tolerate one drop of sauerkraut juice mixed in 4 ounces of water every third day. It may take some trial and error to help you determine the rate of increase that works for your child, and there's no such thing as too slow if it's what works for your kid.

Detox reactions

Detox reactions are incredibly confusing, because they can appear randomly as their body is ready to "deal with" a layer of toxicity. They're easiest to spot shortly after a detox bath, juicing, or other detox strategy has been used. A detox reaction happens when any toxin in the body gets dislodged and overwhelms the body's capability to release it quickly. Your child might experience temporary unpleasant symptoms from this release.

In many children, the detox pathways of the liver, kidneys, skin, and lungs become congested and backed up. If they're not working efficiently and they start dislodging aluminum from their brain, for example, it can't be neutralized and excreted easily by these organs, so it may recirculate, cause symptoms, and then resettle in another part of her body.

A detox reaction can manifest as an increase in a symptom that your child experienced prior to their new diet, like skin issues or self-stimulating, or it may be a new occurrence like headaches, joint aches, itching, an increase in bedwetting or tantrums, or a regression in speech or learning. My skin was my issue, so every time I had a reaction, I would break out with acne.

Some detox reactions are caused by the things that you're doing to aid in detoxification, like juicing, and other times, her detox symptoms will begin when her body gains enough healing energy to start dealing with her backlog of pesticides, vaccine adjuvants, and food additives.

Constipation exacerbates detox reactions, because our number one way to release waste is through our stool. It's not uncommon for children to get very agitated, emotional, have nightmares, or even experience hallucinations or the feeling of a crawling sensation under the skin when they are constipated. These are all signs that toxicity has built up, and you'll notice that they'll subside after a bowel movement.

While it's normal to have a detox reaction on some healing diets, you don't want your child to feel them strongly all the time. A strong reaction tells you you're overdriving their detox pathways. When they have a big reaction, it's a sign that you need to scale back on what you're doing and work back up slowly. It can take a little bit of experimentation to find a manageable pace of detox for your child, and you'll adjust your detox activities accordingly.

Detoxification is something that happens all the time, and you can expect that a detox reaction isn't just a one-time event. It may occur early in the diet, weeks or months into the program, and they may come in waves. Riding these waves through the diet is where I see great gains in health over time. Getting clean on the inside allows your child's body to function optimally all the time.

How to calm a detox reaction

Detox reactions can also be calmed by activated charcoal or modified citrus pectin, like die-off reactions. If you notice a detox reaction from something like juicing or a supplement you're using, a bath may help alleviate the symptoms. If possible, have your child go barefoot outside on grass or dirt for 20 minutes. This grounding of the energy is immensely calming.

To prevent such strong detox reactions, cut down on the amount of detox activities you're doing. This might mean a 10-minute bath instead of 20 minutes, or one ounce of juice instead of a whole glass. Just like with a die-off reaction, you'll use some trial and error to find the activities that are leading to an overall benefit while keeping your life manageable.

Food sensitivity reactions

A food sensitivity will cause a specific reaction that is the same each time, for example, intestinal pain, agitation, spacing out, or sleepiness. The best way to track food sensitivities is through a food journal, because they may be delayed by hours or even a couple of days.

If you've done some type of food allergy or sensitivity testing with your child already, I recommend avoiding those foods that came up reactive for at least three months. After three months of healing, use the Skin Sensitivity Test or the Pulse Test below, with each food as you introduce them. Still have a reaction? Try again in another six weeks. No longer reacting? Add in a small amount and leave a few days in between offering it again.

Sometimes, people discover that they can have a little bit of one of the foods they've been sensitive to and it doesn't cause problems, but if they have it every day or if they have it in large quantities, it does create issues. Your child's body is your guide, so rotate in foods like that if needed.

If your child has had a lifelong allergy to the protein component of a food (IgE reaction), they'll probably need several months or more of healing before they might safely try that food again. I think it's worth testing a tiny amount every six weeks, after *all* their other symptoms have improved a lot. Six or eight months is a common timeframe to try these again, but consult your doctor and only try it when you feel confident in doing so.

Testing food sensitivities for reintroduction

Try one or both of these methods with anything that is a known or suspected allergen or sensitivity. If your child passes the Skin Sensitivity Test and they're old enough to do the Pulse Testing, you'll have more peace of mind when they pass both. Neither of these are 100 percent accurate though, so use your best judgment.

Skin sensitivity testing

The skin sensitivity test works great for babies and small children in particular, but everyone should try it.

- Put a dime-sized drop of a food you want to test on the inside of your child's wrist at bedtime.

- Cover it with a piece of gauze or a piece of cotton or flannel fabric. Use a material that will prevent it from wiping off onto their pajamas or sheets.

- In the morning, uncover it and check the spot. If there's no reaction, you can go ahead and introduce that food, but if there is an angry red reaction, you can consider that an allergy. In that case, you have to leave this food out and try the test again in about three months.

Pulse testing

If your child is old enough to perform this test, it's really helpful and can actually identify subtler sensitivities than a skin test will.

This Pulse Test is a variation on what was discovered by a man named Dr. Coca, whose wife had severe reactions to medications and certain foods, and he noticed that with each reaction her pulse would accelerate. That sparked his theory that when we're allergic to something, it causes a stress response in our body, which raises our pulse. He went on to test this theory with numerous people and all kinds of foods over several years, publishing his findings in a book called *The Pulse Test* in 1956.

I'm sharing the simplified version of The Pulse Test, so you can do it on your child in two and a half minutes, to learn if they have a reaction or intolerance to a particular food or supplement. Yes, it's really that quick!

The Pulse Test

A note of caution: This test might not give you accurate results for people taking a drug that controls their heart rate, like a calcium-channel blocker or a beta-blocker.

Your child must be in a calm state before you begin, because their heart rate needs to be at their normal resting rate.

Step 1. Gather a pen, piece of paper, and a clock or watch with a second hand, or a stopwatch app on your mobile phone. Have your test food within reach when you begin the test.

Step 2. Sit down, take a deep breath, and relax. Start when their heart rate is at a normal pace, not when they've been running around.

Step 3. Determine their starting pulse by counting their heart beat for a full minute. You can use their wrist or neck, as long as you take it at the same place each time. Write down your "before" pulse.

Step 4. Give your child a bite of food and have them chew it, making sure it hits all their taste buds, but tell them not to swallow it. You can also do this with a drink, or a supplement if it's safe to chew on it. Make sure they taste it for at least 30 seconds, because the taste is what informs their central nervous system, which makes the snap judgment on whether this food is safe for them or not. If this food is seen as stressful for their body, their pulse will elevate briefly.

For the most telling results, test one food at a time. You can test a food with multiple ingredients, but to narrow down which is the real culprit, you'll need to test them individually. So, for instance, if you test a nut and squash pancake, are they reacting to the type of nut, squash, ghee, honey, salt, or a spice?

Step 5. Take their pulse for one full minute again while they hold the food in their mouth, and write down the "after" pulse.

An increase of four or more beats is considered the result of a stressful reaction. For those with Type O Blood, an increase of three or more is considered a stressful reaction (some of us are just more sensitive than others.) The bigger the pulse change, the more stressful their body considers this food. I've seen reactions with an increase of 10 or 20 beats per minute.

If your child has a stressful reaction to a food, leave it out for about six weeks. Allow more healing to happen on the diet, and then you can try the Pulse Test again to see if their reaction has changed.

Step 6. Have them spit out the food you're testing if you plan to test another food right away; otherwise, they may have a continued reaction if they swallow the bite. You can do the Pulse Test with as many things as you'd like, as long as you wait for their pulse to return to their "before" rate prior to testing the next food.

If they reacted to a certain food and you want to test another one right away, it helps to have them rinse their mouth out with filtered water and then spit the water out. Then, wait about two minutes and retest their pulse to see if it has returned to its starting rate. If it hasn't, wait another couple of minutes and try again. It doesn't usually take very long.

Note: you must take a full one-minute pulse each time. Taking a fifteen-second pulse and multiplying it by four won't work, because the variation in your pulse can happen at any time during that minute. I've had experiences where my pulse feels nice and steady, and about halfway through the minute, my pulse rate jumps very suddenly.

Digestive reactions

Digestive reactions are typically periodic and temporary, like reflux or loose stools once or twice in a row. Things like this happen from time to time, and it's nothing to worry over. If your child has a lot of gas, most often it's the *prior meal* that caused it. Every meal sends a propulsion reflex down the digestive tract, so gas in the bowel may be released when they eat the *next meal*.

If your child has consistent digestive issues, the next chapter will help you determine if you need supplements to address their issue.

CHAPTER 7: HOW TO KNOW IF YOU NEED SUPPLEMENTS

Supplements might already be part of the plan you're following. If that's the case, you can skip right over this section. I'll discuss what symptoms to look for that indicate digestive support supplements may be useful for your child, along with recommendations on how to use them. This is great information to bring to your child's doctor if you feel these will be useful. Your pediatrician may also prefer to run tests and recommend specific supplements.

With any healing diet, be sure to buy supplements that are free of allergens like wheat, corn, and soy, and are free of fillers and additives like colors, flavors, and sweeteners.

Probiotics

There are hundreds of types of beneficial bacteria that live in the gut and only a small percentage that we've figured out how to put into capsules. That's why fermented foods are important on most gut healing protocols. When it comes to probiotics that you can get as supplements, there are three main types to look for:

Lactobacillus and Bifidobacterium. These are the most common types of probiotics, and you'll see that there are many strains of both Lactobacillus and Bifidobacterium, often paired in a formula together. Lactobacillus is mostly transient, which means that when we take them they go into our digestive system, do their job, and then become part of our stool. We need to take these in on a regular basis because they don't stick around. Bifidobacterium mostly reside in the colon, so they're an important part of our stool. These two are also the most common types that you'll find in fermented foods like sauerkraut and yogurt.

Probiotic yeasts, like Saccharomyces Boulardii. Probiotic yeast can do battle with the opportunistic yeasts, such as Candida Albicans, that might be over-represented in your child's gut right now. If you suspect that your child has Candida overgrowth, giving him Saccharomyces Boulardii for a period of time can be helpful in getting Candida back into balance. Saccharomyces Boulardii is also a transient probiotic, so it will only be at work while you're taking it. Probiotic yeasts are also found in kefir, both dairy and coconut-based.

Soil-based organisms. Soil-based organisms are also known as spore-forming organisms. They are a whole different class, because they are considered native to our digestive system. In the past, our ancestors worked in organic agriculture and animal husbandry. Just like the name sounds, soil-based organisms are in the soil and would be inhaled as dust and eaten on slightly dirty food.

Nowadays, our food is so sanitized that we really don't come into contact with this type of bacteria very often. If we're born with healthy gut flora and we never take antibiotics, we have these types of bacteria taking care of us in our gut: living, procreating, and carrying on happily forever.

Unfortunately, most of our kids aren't born this way, and when they take antibiotics, these guys get wiped out. The good news about soil-based organisms is that we can reestablish a good colony and we don't need to take them forever. Taking these for a few months, or interspersing them a couple times a week with other types of probiotics, is a great way to get them reestablished. I've found that soil-based probiotics are the best ones to start with in cases of constipation, small intestine bacterial overgrowth (SIBO), and autism or other sensory processing disorders.

No matter what type of probiotic you try with your child, realize that different types and strains will affect them differently. For example, you may see no reaction whatsoever from a Lactobacillus species, but when you take Saccharomyces Boulardii, they may wet the bed or develop a patch of eczema from a die-off reaction.

Anytime you try something that's new and different, open the capsule to start with just a pinch to ¼ of a capsule. If your child has a die-off reaction, wait until it passes, and then start again with a smaller amount.

To cover your bases with each of these types of probiotic, I suggest rotating through different probiotics at least every three to six months, in addition to eating a variety of fermented foods.

Recommended probiotic dosages for all ages

Different probiotics have the best effect at different dosages, and there are different recommended doses of probiotics based on a person's age. On top of that, we have at least three types of probiotic that are in capsules: the Lactobacillus-bifidobacteria strains, probiotic yeasts, and soil-based bacteria.

Here are some guidelines for how much of each type to take based on age, but keep in mind that these are *general recommendations* and everybody is different. With any new probiotic, start with a small amount and work up slowly. That can mean as slow as a pinch once a week. On the other hand, some people benefit from much higher doses, and the only way to find that out is to listen to your own intuition and use your child's symptoms as your guide.

In a child, die-off can show up as a change in behavior, disturbed sleep, bed wetting, skin rash, reduced learning ability or eye contact, or an increase in any of their usual symptoms or issues.

Infant probiotics are useful for newborn babies and very small children, especially:

- If mom has digestive issues or an autoimmune condition.

- If the baby was born by C-section.

- If the child has already taken a course of antibiotics.

- If the child has undergone another type of medical intervention.

Bifidobacteria infantis is the most common type that you'll find for babies, but some formulations include other strains that are prevalent in a healthy infant gut.

To give probiotics to your baby:

- If you're nursing, just put a slight dusting on your nipples at feeding time once or twice a day.

- Add a little pinch of the probiotic powder in with the formula you're making.

- Or, if they're eating solids already, sprinkle a pinch on cooled foods.

A therapeutic dose for probiotics is very individual, so take these as general recommendations. Please be aware that these are the full doses, and you may need to start out with a much smaller dose and build up slowly.

Lacto-bifido strains of probiotics

Age	Billion bacterial cells per day
Infant to 12 months	1-2 billion
1-2 years old	2-4 billion
2-4 years old	4-8 billion
4-10 years old	8-12 billion
10-12 years old	12-15 billion
12-16 years old	15-20 billion
17 years to adult	20-25 billion

Once you reach your therapeutic dose, you should maintain that level for at least six months.

Saccharomyces Boulardii (probiotic yeast)

Age	Billion bacterial cells per day
0-2 years old	Homemade kefir
3-5 years old	1 billion
6-11 years old	2 billion
12-17 years old	3-4 billion
18 years and adult	4-5 billion

Work up to these recommendations, then stay at this level for three to four months, after which time you can gradually reduce to none. Always combine S. Boulardii with other probiotics, so the S. Boulardii doesn't dominate the gut.

Soil-based or spore-forming strains

Age	Billion bacterial cells per day
2-5 years old	5 billion
6-11 years old	12 billion
12 years old-adult	25 billion

Soil-based strains are indicated for short-term use of three months or less. Once you've taken a "course" of it, you don't need to continue. You may take them again after you take antibiotics, or have recovered from a severe gut infection.

I recommend that you rotate through different types of probiotics to get the best effect. There *can* be too much of a good thing, and if your body becomes acclimated to one type for a long period of time, it isn't as helpful as having variety. Of course, you should be complementing your capsule probiotics with a variety of fermented foods as part of our daily diet too.

Stomach acid support

Stomach acid support may be needed if your child experiences acid reflux, burping a lot during or right after a meal, if they have an aversion to meat, or feel like food sits like a rock in their stomach. The stomach sits on the left side, under the rib cage, about where the ribs meet in the middle. If your kid says they have a tummy ache, ask them to point to the area to see if it's the stomach or lower on the abdomen, in the intestines.

For boosting stomach acid in young children, I recommend using liquid herbal bitters, a teaspoon of apple cider vinegar mixed in enough water to drink it quickly, or sauerkraut juice at the beginning of each meal, or even 10-15 minutes before the meal. Bitter tastes stimulate our own gastric secretions, priming the stomach for food. Components in cabbage are healing to the stomach lining and gently stimulate stomach acid production.

You may also find a supplemental formula with co-factors to building stomach acid, like zinc carnosine, B vitamins, and pepsin (the enzyme activated by hydrochloric acid or HCl). I prefer to avoid directly using HCl until we've tried the above suggestions *and* the child is at a developmental stage to easily swallow a bit of powdered supplement, or a pill.

For older children suffering with reflux and excessive burping, you may try supplementing *Betaine HCl (hydrochloride)* with co-factors.

- Start with a pinch of the powder (or small amount of crushed tablet) mixed with the first mouthfuls of food.

- Gradually increase the amount to a third or a half capsule per meal; whichever amount creates a change in their symptoms.

HCl should never be taken by children on pain medications, corticosteroids, anti-inflammatories, or other medications.

Digestive enzymes

Digestive Enzymes help break down foods in the small intestine, and I find them especially helpful for bloating. To get the best results, look for a type with a broad spectrum that includes enzymes for carbohydrates, fats, and protein.

Specific enzymes that break down phenols, salicylates, gluten, casein, lactose, histamine, and other food compounds have been developed and are available from a growing number of supplement companies. These can be useful in cases of severe intolerance to those food compounds, when they are taken with every meal and snack.

For example, if your child has severe burning with urination, eczema, and red ears, these are signs of phenol sensitivity and an enzyme that digests phenols can bring a relief for him. Once his gut heals, these supplements can be discontinued.

Fat digestion support

If your child experiences nausea, vomiting, or other digestive upset with fatty meals, or if you see undigested fats in their stool, a bile thinning supplement can support proper fat digestion. Common ingredients are beetroot and black radish. In addition, have your child drink one to two ounces of beet kvass (recipe in Resources) or eat a small serving of beets before each meal. These supplements and foods can also help with constipation.

In severe cases, you may try an ox bile supplement. Crush the tablet or open the capsule to add a small sprinkle in a bite of food with any meal that contains fat.

Other supplements

Magnesium. Many children who experience constipation, leg cramps, or anxiety find great relief with magnesium supplements. I most often recommend magnesium glycinate, because it's easy to digest and absorb, doesn't cause diarrhea, and isn't habit forming. Other forms can be used as well, but whichever form you choose, make sure it's pure and that you give it to your child daily to address magnesium deficiency, not periodically in large amounts like a laxative.

Normal daily recommended intake is[4]:

Persons	U.S. (mg)	Canada (mg)
Infants birth to 3 years	40 to 80	20–50
Children 4 to 6 years	120	65

Children 7 to 10 years	170	100–135
Adolescent and adult males	270–400	130–250
Adolescent and adult females	280–300	135–210

I find that, based on symptoms and blood test results, up to double these doses can be needed and safe when you are overcoming a deficiency. Find the brands I recommend on the Picky Eater Approved page of my website.

---

4 http://www.mayoclinic.org/drugs-supplements/magnesium-supplement-oral-route

CHAPTER 8: DETOX YOUR HOME

In my practice, a focus on detoxification returns continued benefits long after your child is tolerating nourishing foods.

Kids on the autism spectrum and those with other severe disorders are often more toxic than we realize. Even their digestive systems become a source of toxicity. Harmful microbes that are overgrowing in their intestines add their toxic metabolic waste products to our kids' bodies. On top of that, our children absorb toxicity from the outside, too, from things they breathe, put on their skin, and ingest.

Natural detoxification can take several years, and you can't rush through it. Even when you do a significant amount of detox and you remove as many toxic products from your child's life as possible, they'll always be exposed to pollution in the air they breathe, man-made materials they touch, and the building materials they come into contact with every day. Detoxification is an ongoing process that needs to be supported with a steady supply of nutrients, to help your child's detoxification organs continually do their best work.

Die-off and detox reactions aren't something you can "power through." When there's a reaction, your child's symptoms tell you their detoxification system organs—the liver, kidneys, lungs, and skin—are overloaded and can't efficiently process out what's been released. You must go slow enough to find the sweet spot where you know it's working, but life is manageable. Safely removing toxins from the body is a delicate balance. Trust that your child's body knows how to do this, when it's supported with nutrients and other gentle processes that allow it to detoxify in its own way.

There are many ways to support detoxification, and your chosen diet may have specific detoxification recommendations, so please implement them. The simplest and most important place to start is with reducing daily toxin exposure by switching to non-toxic body cleaning and household products. This makes an incredible contribution to healing in the long run!

Detox your home

Reducing daily toxin exposure, coupled with nutrient-dense foods, will allow your child's detoxification system to work through their backlog of toxicity over time.

The general toxic load we carry is due to the fact that anything toxic we eat, breathe, touch, or put on our skin absorbs very quickly and adds work to our natural detox system. So, the less we come in to contact with those substances, the less our bodies have to deal with. This means eliminating or reducing exposure to toxic soaps, shampoo, toothpaste, household cleaners, candles, air fresheners, detergents, and fabric softener, as well as new paint, carpets, and furniture. Be wary of anything that is scented or has a smell that is made from anything other than essential oils.

By minimizing the chemicals your child is exposed to at home, their body will be able to heal much more quickly. You'll find many simple body care and household cleaning recipes, online and in books, that are very safe and use non-toxic ingredients like coconut oil, baking soda, white vinegar, lemon, and essential oils.

If do-it-yourself recipes aren't your thing, you can find non-toxic, premade products, but you must learn to read the ingredient labels on every product you bring into your home. Claims made on packaging, such as "organic" or "natural" hold no legal meaning when it comes to cosmetics, body care, and cleaning products.

Fortunately, there's a non-profit called Environment Working Group, that makes reading labels easy to understand and also makes a phone app where you can scan barcodes! To find out how your body care products rate for safety, look each of them up on the Environmental Working Group's "Skin Deep" website [see Resources]. Use their household product section [see Resources] to look up cleaning products. When you need to buy something new, you can use their lists of the safest products.

Here are specific areas to switch out in your home:

- Hand soap.

  » A plain castile soap is a safer option.

- Shampoo and conditioner.

  » Most children can use "no poo." Simply scrub their hair with only water, or a small amount of baking soda made into a paste.

  » 50/50 diluted apple cider vinegar/water is a simple conditioning rinse.

  » It takes about 30 days for your child's hair to adjust to this and it may look greasy in the meantime. If you're using baking soda and your child has hair longer than their shoulders, or especially thick hair, you may need a natural shampoo and conditioner, since baking soda will take longer to rinse out.

- Body wash and bubble baths.

  » Unscented castile soap is a safer option, but only use it on areas that are actually dirty. Washing with water is enough for most areas and is less disturbing to healthy skin bacteria.

- Baby wipes.

- Toothpaste, floss, and mouthwash.

  » Mixing up a paste of baking soda and olive oil, with a drop or two of their favorite essential oil for flavor, is safe.

- Lip balm.

- Lotions.

  » Try plain coconut oil, beef tallow, or other natural fats or oils.

- Sunscreen.

  » Look for physical (non-chemical) sunscreens without nanoparticles.

- Anything advertised as "anti-bacterial."

- Dish soap.

  » In addition to soaking our hands in this, the fragrance pollutes the air and residue may be left on dishes.

- Dishwasher detergent and rinse aid.

  » Fragrance pollutes the air and residue may be left on dishes.

- Kitchen counter sprays and wipes.

  » White vinegar or Thieves Household Cleaner in a spray bottle is a simple alternative.

- Laundry detergent.

- Fabric softener.

  » This is one of the most toxic products in most homes and adds to terrible air quality in your house. Try wool balls.

- Household cleaners.

- Bathroom scrubs.

  » Baking soda works as well.

- Window cleaner.

- Carpet deodorizers or cleaning solutions.

- Candles.

- Air fresheners, plug-ins, and sprays.

  » These basically just spew out cancer-causing chemicals. They are my biggest pet peeve! Use pure essential oils in a diffuser instead.

- Pet care products.

  » They are tracking these all over your home, and your kids are probably snuggling up with them.

- Lawn chemicals, pesticides, and fertilizers.

  » Your children and pets are poisoned by these, and they track them in the house too!

- Any products that you or other household members use that will be in the air or rub on to your child through typical contact, like perfume, make-up, and hair styling products.

This is a long list, and it's not something you'll switch in one day. Just work through it one area at a time, and within a few months your whole home will be a non-toxic showplace. Then you'll begin to notice how toxic every other place you go is!

Find out what I'm currently using to clean my home on the Picky Eater Approved page of my website.

Air purification

If your child has any type of allergies, eczema, or asthma, make sure you take extra steps to improve your indoor air quality.

Switching out your body care and cleaning products will go a long way, but you should also consider an air purifier in your child's bedroom and any other area they spend a lot of time in. Houseplants can help clean the air too, so plan to have lots of them around your house! Your child may enjoy picking them out and caring for them.

You can also ask to bring plants or an air purifier to their classroom at school. Unfortunately, our schools are usually a source of toxic air from cleaning agents and building materials. Make an effort to detoxify that environment too because your child spends a lot of time there.

Mold

Molds are some of the most harmful substances your child may be in contact with, and a body can't heal when it's continually assaulted by mold. If you have mold in your home or your child's school, *it must be remediated or you must move as soon as possible.*

If your child has allergies, especially anaphylactic, or any chronic immune or neurological condition, this is an immediate priority.

You will see an incredible leap in healing once this is addressed!

For more information and resources on mold, please see the Picky Eater Approved page of my website.

CHAPTER 9: WHAT TO DO EVERYDAY

One of the biggest concerns that parents face after they've started a healing protocol, is how to keep on top of everything that needs to be done every day.

It's a lifestyle adjustment, and some of the things take time to make a habit of. If it isn't realistic for you to do everything every day, don't. Just commit 100 percent to the food right now. You can add the other parts later, or sporadically, to see what difference they make. Some healing protocol is better than no healing protocol!

Make yourself a spreadsheet, chart, or whiteboard that you can hang up in the kitchen and interact with every day. Charts meant for teachers work great for this. You can write in the daily activities along one side and the kids' names or days of the week on the other, then check off each item throughout the day.

Key points to remember:

- Variety is key in the long run. Variation covers more nutritional bases and leads to less food sensitivity.

- Don't rush! Results don't happen overnight for most families. Move through your plan slowly so you can easily tell which foods don't work right now. You'll get to all of it.

- Don't make fancy food. Keep it simple. Homemade food is delicious, so let the good quality ingredients speak for themselves.

- You can make a "formula" for yourself to make meals simpler. An example is soup for breakfast and meat casserole for dinner, with those leftovers as the next day's lunch. With this idea, you can have a soup pot or a couple of slow cookers going each day, then just change out the meat, veggies, and seasonings for variety.

- Keep a simple diary. The best type is the one that you'll jot things down in daily. Your memory isn't good enough to pick up the small patterns without reviewing something written down.

- Be creative and flexible. It's about figuring out what works with *your* kid.

CHAPTER 10:
TROUBLESHOOTING ISSUES

Here, you'll learn the most common issues that will come up on healing diets, what they mean, and what to do about them.

There are many, many natural remedies out there, so if ideas from this section aren't working for you, do more research to find other things to try. Everyone is an individual, so what works perfectly for one family might not work at all for you.

Coming down with a cold, flu, or other illness in the beginning of a new diet is perfectly normal. The immune system is trying out its new power. Expect another bout of illness (ear infection, sore throat, urinary tract infection), or behavior or learning regression about two to three months into the new diet. You will then experience waves like this every so often for the first couple of years, as your child's body retraces through old illness and deals with them for good, or brings up toxins and discharges them. If you're curious, can afford it, and want to monitor this through Hair Mineral Tissue Analysis testing every three months, it's quite interesting.

Before you decide on any remedy, take a deep breath and ask yourself, "Is this a true problem, or am I panicking under stress?" So many times, parents have an extreme reaction to something that's a one-time thing. One episode of diarrhea or vomiting is not a true problem. Two to three days of this might be. If your kid has a high fever in conjunction with diarrhea and/or vomiting, they may actually be sick and should be taken to your local pediatric naturopath, homeopath, or other doctor to be safe.

Bedwetting

Bedwetting that increases or begins again on a healing diet is a sign of a detox reaction. Cut down the fermented foods and probiotic capsules by 50 percent, and see if that makes a difference within a couple of days. If not, cut down by another 50 percent again. Work back up as slowly as you need to keep this from recurring.

Constipation

It's common for your child's bowel movements to change early on a new diet. Whether constipation has been an ongoing issue with your child, or if it's set in with the change in food, there are many natural options you can try to improve his bowel movements. In some kids, grains and fiber-rich foods, or food sensitivities, are inflaming the intestinal lining. His body may have been trying to rid itself of these quickly, causing loose bowel movements, and removing them can result in constipation.

Since constipation is a slowing-down in the digestive tract, it's something that takes a while to completely overcome if it's been an ongoing issue. There can be many reasons why your child is constipated, because several factors go into creating a perfect bowel movement. The areas that you'll need to work on to correct his bowel movements in the long run are:

- Hydration.

- Good bacteria balance.

- Mineral balance.

- Optimal thyroid function.

- Proper fat digestion (bile provides the lubricant for our stool to pass easily).

- Some fiber.

- Good stomach acid to set the stage for proper digestion all the way through.

- Functional Migrating Motor Complex (MMC), which can be slowed or stopped in cases of Small Intestine Bacterial Overgrowth (SIBO), or with injury that affects the vagal nerve connection.

I always look "north" to see what may have gone wrong prior to the colon. We expect that constipation originates in the colon, but that's often not the case. While you're working on all of the areas above, here are some ideas you can try for constipation relief right now. Just be aware that these are remedies and not the solution. You have to do the work above.

Hydrate. Have your child drink eight to twelve ounces of room temperature or warm water first thing in the morning, with half a teaspoon of natural sea salt dissolved in it. This rehydrates her body and provides a signal to the stretch receptors in the stomach, which triggers food elsewhere in the digestive system to move on down the line.

Carrot, celery, or cucumber juice. Add fresh-pressed juices, particularly carrot-cucumber juice mixed with either cod liver oil or olive oil, before bedtime. These veggies are higher in potassium, which helps to retain water in the bowel. There are certain fast-moving waves that go through the digestive tract while your child sleeps at night (MMC), so this remedy can lead to an easy bowel movement the next morning.

Beet kvass. Beet kvass is a fermented beet beverage that adds probiotics and bile-thinning components present in beets. Start small with this, because it can cause a die-off reaction. If fat digestion is an issue for your child, drinking one to two ounces of beet kvass before each meal can help thin her bile, and keep that meal moving through at a steady pace. Cooked or raw beets are also helpful.

Increase veggies. It's so common for picky kids to not eat enough vegetable fiber (which also happens to be common in adults). Load up your child's plate with veggies or sneak them into everything by adding minced or pureed veggies to soups, stews, and ground meats.

Soil-based probiotics. Soil-based probiotics are a type that many people haven't taken, and it's important to repopulate this native flora. I've found that for many people, using Klaire Labs BioSpora or MegaSporeBiotic for a few months can help immensely with constipation.

Magnesium. Many people recommend magnesium oxide or magnesium citrate for constipation. I think these are okay, but those forms do draw water into the bowel and can force a loose bowel movement. If you do this often as a laxative, your child's body can get used to that influx of water into the colon and can become dependent upon it. I prefer to use the magnesium glycinate form, because it's easy to absorb in a damaged gut, and it doesn't draw water to the bowel. Instead, it allows the magnesium to be used in all of the enzymes binding sites, as well as the smooth muscles that need to relax for bowel movements. Start with about 100mg, and add 100mg at a time, until you find the dose that works for your child. It's best to divide larger doses over the day. This isn't an overnight fix, but if magnesium deficiency is part of why your child is constipated, you'll find the level that allows them to have an easy bowel movement every day.

High-fat dairy. Fat stimulates the release of bile, which is the lubricant for the stool. If your child has been eating dairy but you've been focusing on higher-protein types like low-fat yogurt, cheese, and kefir, switch to sour cream and full-fat yogurts. For some people, dairy in general is constipating, so you may want to try a few weeks without it to see if that makes a difference for your kid.

Castor oil packs over the liver or colon. Castor oil can penetrate the tissues of the body and can help either decongest the liver if that's the source of constipation, or loosen dried masses of feces from the colon if that's where the issue is.

To Make a Castor Oil Pack, You'll Need:

- Castor oil.

- Three layers of organic wool, cotton flannel, or cotton towel. Make sure this is big enough to cover the whole area you're placing it on.

- Plastic wrap cut one to two inches larger than the flannel. You can also "wrap" your child in cling wrap, cut a plastic bag, or use an old, thin towel or blanket (the oil will seep through fabric).

- Hot water bottle.

- Old clothes and sheets (castor oil will stain clothing and bedding).

- Container with lid to soak the flannel and to store the pack in, to be reused later.

To Use:

- Place the flannel in the container. Soak it in castor oil so that it's saturated but not dripping.

- Place the pack over the body part you're working on.

- Cover with plastic or layers of old towels.

- Place the hot water bottle over the pack. Leave it on for 45-60 minutes. Have your child rest or nap while the pack is in place.

- After you remove the pack, you can wash the skin with water and a little bit of baking soda to remove the oil.

- Store the pack in the covered container in the refrigerator. Each pack may be reused up to 25-30 times.

- Repeat this three nights in a row, then take three nights off, three nights on, and so on.

Enema. Enemas are the last thing on everybody's list to try, but there is no better relief from constipation than an enema. It's one of those things that sounds really weird until you do it, and then you realize that it's just not that big of a deal, and the relief it provides is wonderful! A water enema can fill the colon and allow the softening of any stool that is hardened or stuck to the sides of the colon, so that it can be permanently released.

Enemas are very safe for babies, children, and adults, and are extremely helpful for reducing the toxic load in the body, relieving constipation, removing fecal compaction from the bowel, introducing probiotics directly into the bowel, cleansing the liver, and healing hemorrhoids. Enemas were routinely used in hospitals until the invention of medicated suppositories, which are quicker to administer for the staff.

I *highly recommend* that you perform an enema on yourself (even if you aren't constipated) to get over your fears about them before you perform one on your child. She will feel your anxiety about the procedure and will feel anxious herself.

To prepare, set out towels in the bathtub or on the floor near the toilet. Have a video, book, or toy to keep your child's attention.

Supplies:

- An enema bag, bucket, or bulb syringe as indicated by age below*.

- Stainless steel cooking pot.

- Pure water (chlorinated water should be boiled for 10 minutes to release this).

- Olive oil or other natural lubricant.

*A see-through enema bag or an enema bucket is nicer, but an old-fashioned type that doubles as a hot water bottle can be used.

Directions:

1. Bring the appropriate amount of water to a boil, then turn it off and let it cool to body temperature. (See amounts by age below).

2. Fill your syringe, bag, or bucket and then test the temperature with your finger. It should be the same temperature as a baby's bottle (tepid). It's safer to have it too cold than too warm. Never use hot or steaming water; body temperature is good. Add more cool filtered water if necessary.

3. Lubricate the nozzle with olive oil, coconut oil, or a vitamin E capsule. Avoid petroleum-based lubricants.

4. Have your child lie on their right side, with their knees pulled up toward their belly (this straightens the last part of the colon for easier insertion), and gently insert the nozzle into the rectum a few inches. At the correct angle, it will insert without resistance. If you feel like you're bumping into something, pull back, take a breath, and try again at a slightly different angle. Never use force.

5. Let the water flow in, but clamp the tubing off as soon as there is the slightest amount of discomfort or fullness. This is typically a gas bubble, and the sensation will usually

pass within a few seconds. Then, you can release the clamp to allow more water to flow in.

6. When all the water is in, tell your child to hold the water in as you remove the tip. In a baby or toddler, you can hold their bum cheeks together.

7. It may be helpful to gently massage your child's colon from the bottom left hipbone, across the top of their abdomen, and down to their right hip bone. This can help the water move through the entire space.

8. Have them retain the enema as long as they can. 12 to 15 minutes is ideal. Turning over to the other side or moving to hands and knees can sometimes be more comfortable. Find what works. Sometimes, there will be an immediate urgency to get rid of it and that is fine. It helps to clean the stool out of the lower colon so that next time around they can hold more for longer. Never force your child to retain it if they feel they can't.

9. Move to the toilet and allow everything to come out. If they don't feel "done," it can help to massage their abdomen from the bottom right, up across the top, and down the left side, tracing the natural exit path of the colon. It is natural to release a lot of it, then sit there for a few minutes, and then release more. It can take 10 to 15 minutes to feel "done." If your child feels done, but very little came out, they've absorbed this water because they were dehydrated.

10. For stubborn constipation, you can repeat this process until the water runs out clear. It can take a few enemas to loosen compacted feces from the walls of the colon.

11. When you have finished your session, wash the tip, rinse out the bag, and hang it up to dry. Periodically run boiling water, peroxide, or another comparable antimicrobial agent through the empty bag to discourage mold growth when not in use.

For babies and small children up to two years of age, use enemas in cases of constipation only if the child has not passed stool for two days or more. Use a bulb syringe enema kit; the usual sizes of bulb syringes available are 50 ml (about 2 oz) or 100 ml (about 4 oz). Fill the syringe with warm filtered water (about body temperature), lubricate the nozzle and the anus of the baby with coconut oil, olive oil, or butter, then insert the nozzle into the anus and gently squeeze the bulb, letting the water into the bowel. Remove the nozzle, hold the bottom of the child closed while gently massaging the tummy for a minute or two, and then let the baby empty the bowel. Use only clean filtered or bottled water.

For children from three to five years old, use a bulb syringe or an enema bag or bucket. For this age group, you can add some probiotic to the enema water, about 1-2 billion live cells per enema, preferably from the Bifidobacteria group.

For children older than five, use an enema bag or bucket, because the syringe bulb won't provide enough water. You can add probiotics to the enema water, about 3-4 billion live cells per enema, preferably from the Bifidobacteria group. You can also add a ½ teaspoon of natural salt per every quart of water used, to help them retain the water for a few minutes.

Always discontinue enemas if they have any adverse reaction, and discuss it with your healthcare practitioner.

Colon hydrotherapy. If your child has a long history of constipation, and especially if you're nervous about doing enemas at home, I recommend going to a colon hydrotherapy center and having your child try a few treatments there. Colon hydrotherapy is different from an enema, in that it gently cleanses the entire length of the colon and softens masses that may be stuck to the walls of the colon, so that you can be rid of them forever. A colon hydrotherapist may also help you understand how to do enemas at home if you feel unsure about it.

Chronic constipation doesn't resolve overnight. You can get relief by having a bowel movement using one of these remedies, but you have to work on the underlying systems that are involved in order to have perfect bowel movements on a very consistent basis. As your child's digestion heals and they become completely nourished through diet and other healing activities, their bowel movements will become more regular.

Eczema and other skin conditions

One of the most common issues affecting children with digestive problems is eczema. It often improves when people remove their allergens in the first place, and then flares a bit periodically as toxins are discharged through the skin. Over time, diet and detoxification will completely remove symptoms of eczema and dry skin. In the meantime, there are several topical remedies you can use. Different things work for different people, so expect a little trial and error to find out what soothes your child's skin.

Don't use soap or other chemicals on the skin and hair, because they wash off protective oils and dry out the skin. They also wash off the habitat for your beneficial skin flora, which leaves your skin open to invasion by pathogens. Wash only with water, in order to maintain the protective oils and the skin's pH balance.

Detoxification baths can be very helpful. Baths can be very effective in gently removing toxins from the body, because the skin takes in some nutrients from the bath and releases toxins into the bath water.

Baths can be strongly detoxifying, so start with less additive, cooler water, and less time in the bath if your child is very toxic, sensitive, or has had a detox reaction to a prior bath. Work up to baths that last 20-40 minutes.

You may use baths daily, alternating through the following additions:

Epsom salts (½ cup): You can find these at any drug store or online. In an Epsom salt bath, you absorb magnesium, which is needed for detoxification and muscle relaxation, as well as sulfate, which is critical for the liver to process toxins out.

Apple cider vinegar (½ cup): Apple cider vinegar (ACV) contains a large complement of minerals that the skin will absorb.

Baking soda (½ cup): Baking soda can be especially soothing for itchy skin conditions, such as eczema, and has anti-fungal properties.

Sea Salt (½ cup): Natural sea salts contain a large variety of trace minerals that can be absorbed by the skin.

Seaweed powder (1/4 cup): This is hard to find locally and tends to be very expensive when it's labeled as a special bath additive. I prefer to purchase bulk seaweed powders online, which are much cheaper. This is a really wonderful addition, so don't skip it; the body can absorb so many trace minerals from seaweed powder in the bath. Using seaweed powder in the bath smells like bathing in a tide pool. You'll have to clean your bathtub afterward, so you may only do this one once a week.

Clays (¼ to ½ cup): Clays are particularly known for their ability to remove toxic metals from the air, water, and soil because of their unusual structure of "pores" (channels and holes), that allows them to absorb huge amounts of contaminant materials. There are many types of clays, and each one has a different chemical composition and purpose.

A variety of brands of bath additives are out there, and you can find my current favorites on the Picky Eater Approved page of my website.

No bathtub, no problem

If you don't have a bathtub, find that detox baths are too strong for your child, or having your child sit in the bath each night isn't feasible, foot baths offer an alternative. Our feet have large pores, so you can add the bath additive to a smaller basin of water to get the benefit of the bath.

You can also use this method for things like a stubborn patch of eczema on an elbow, for example. Have her soak her arm in a small basin of water with baking soda when she doesn't have the time for a full bath.

After the bath, apply one of the following:

- A thin layer of homemade yogurt, kefir, or sour cream to inoculate the skin with beneficial bacteria.

- A pure oil like jojoba or food-grade sesame oil, olive oil, or coconut oil.

For severe eczema patches, try overnight applications of raw honey or seaweed powder.

- The first night, apply Manuka honey thickly over the eczema, then cover with cling wrap or a piece of flannel covered with cling wrap and taped on. Have your child sleep like this. In the morning, wash the honey off and apply one of the above cultured foods or oils.

- The second night, try an application of seaweed powder made by mixing two tablespoons of seaweed powder with a small amount of hot water to form a paste. Apply this just like the honey and follow up the same way.

Swimming in the sea and sunbathing do wonders for eczema, psoriasis, and other skin problems, so engage in these activities as often as you can.

For diaper rashes, apply homemade kefir or kefir cream (sour cream made with kefir culture) at every diaper change. Coconut oil can also be used.

Extreme fatigue or "zombie" behavior

Extreme fatigue, or being so tired that your child is like a zombie, is very common in the early days of a dramatically different diet. Expect to see this when your child has been fasting (not eating) for a couple of days. Let them rest. Don't try to get them to do anything. They'll work through it. Just be mindful that they're not experiencing dangerously low blood sugar levels. See Chapter 6 for more details.

Hunger

Parents often remark that they can't believe how much their kids are eating on a healing diet, and they wonder if it's normal. They're especially amazed when it's their picky kids who are now ravenous.

There are four reasons your child is always hungry on a new diet:

1. *You just started the diet.* Once your kid starts eating, it's common for them to feel ravenous. Their body is *finally* getting the nourishment that it needs to heal, and it says, "Keep it coming." This is usually most applicable to meats. You might feel like they're eating so much meat that it can't possibly be healthy, and it never seems like it's going to end. This is really common for two or three months. Then one day, it's like a switch flips, and all the sudden, they feel satiated with a normal portion of protein at each meal.

2. *They're not eating enough fat.* This is usually more apparent when they've been on a new diet for a few months. If your kids are constantly hungry or feel like they need snacks every hour or two, they're not eating enough fat. Increase the amount of added fat (or total food) until they feel satiated for at least four hours until the next meal.

3. *Your kids are growing.* When your kids are past the toddler phase, there are so many growth spurts. I hear from parents all the time that their kids eat just as much food as they do and sometimes more. As long as your kids are eating whole, nutrient-dense food, just go with it. When we give our kids natural, healthy options, they become very instinctual about the amounts and types of foods that they need to eat at any given time.

4. *Their microbes have cravings.* If your kids are always hungry but their cravings are for the carbohydrates like fruit, honey, and sweet things, that's more likely to be their microbes talking. A big part of any gut-healing diet is to get those bugs back in balance. Focus on fermented and savory foods, and limit the sweeter things to help them do that. You *do* want to make sure that you're including enough starches like winter squashes or a little bit of fruit to keep their glucose needs met. Occasionally, people feel hungry or out of balance because they're eating too few carbohydrates, which can be accidental. Be mindful of this to see if adding a few more carbs helps them remain satiated or leads them to more compulsive carb cravings.

When they're hungry, they need to eat a full meal. Snacks are to hold your child over when they truly can't eat a whole meal, like during travel or on a hike. Don't let them graze all day, because this sets them up for blood sugar dysregulation and provides a constant source of food in the intestinal tract for microbial overgrowth. As much as possible, honor your child's hunger by giving them nutrient-filled meals with plenty of fat and protein to keep them satisfied in between. This can also help with needed weight gain.

Oxalates

Oxalates are a naturally-occurring chemical component of plant foods that we eat, and that are sprayed on crops through pesticides. With a healthy gut, they aren't an issue, but in a leaky gut, they can cause problems, particularly in cases of autism and arthritis.

In a non-leaky human gut, oxalates are degraded by the bacteria oxalobacter formigenes. In a leaky gut or when oxalobacter is low (like after antibiotics), oxalates can be absorbed into the bloodstream rather than being excreted in the stool. In a healthy gut, one to two percent of oxalates are absorbed, but in a leaky gut, as much as 50 percent may be absorbed into the blood. When they're absorbed, oxalates create inflammation, interfere with nutrient absorption, lead to oxidative stress, and can mess with mitochondrial (cell energy) function.

Almonds are often used liberally on grain-free diets, but they're also very high in oxalates, as are several other veggies, nuts, seeds, and fruit. I think this is a major factor that helps to explain why most of the kids with autism I work with don't do well with nuts or seeds for six to eight months.

If you suspect oxalates are an issue for your child, limit them in the diet for a while and observe the symptom improvement. For a more complete list of oxalate-rich foods, check out the Picky Eater Approved page of my website. After a few months of healing, you can try adding in more oxalate-containing foods to see if your child can handle them better.

Vitamin B6 is usually low with oxalate issues, so consider supplementing by building it up slowly or testing to see your child's level. L-lysine is needed for B6's use. The citrate form of minerals also binds to oxalates to help them be removed from the body, so slowly supplementing magnesium or calcium citrate can help as well. Supplementing too much too quickly can exacerbate symptoms, so go super-slow with them.

Red face

Red cheeks, ears, or a flushed look can be due to Histamine Reaction or Phenol Sensitivity, which includes Salicylates.

Histamine is a chemical in the body that sends messages between cells and acts as a mediator in inflammatory and allergic responses. It's present in many foods, especially those that are aged, and in leftovers (which is also aging food). There are certain bacteria and enzymes that degrade histamine, so that we don't have too much of it in the body at once. If these aren't sufficiently present, there can be an overload of histamine in the body, leading to reactions. (See Resources for more info on how to manage these reactions.)

Salicylates are naturally-occurring chemicals that are found in almost all foods, but particularly vegetables, fruits, and nuts. There's an enzyme your child may be deficient in that processes these out, and a leaky gut exacerbates this issue. With phenol issues, you can hybridize the diet you're following with a low salicylate diet (there's no such thing as a "no salicylate diet") while the gut is healing. Peeling and cooking vegetables helps a lot. Healing the gut overcomes this sensitivity in time. (See Resources for more info on how to manage these reactions.)

Eczema can also show up as red patches on the face, but they also have a rough texture.

Regression and tantrums

Regression and tantrums can be caused by a food reaction or a detoxification reaction. With tantrums, you're breaking your child of drug-like foods, and they (their microbes) are not happy to do this! Keep your emotions calm and let them run their course without extra attention. This is part of the process, so be okay with that.

The most common food culprits for regression and tantrums are: fruit, honey, nuts, dairy, gluten, grains, and eggs. Review your food diary for clues on foods that have been introduced or increased in the past couple of weeks. Cut down on probiotics, fermented foods, or other detoxification activities as needed. Of course, regression and tantrums can also be from cheating on the diet with gluten or sweets, so look for that too.

Weight loss

Weight loss at the very beginning is to be expected. Whether your child refuses food in the beginning or not, you should be prepared for this. A thin child eating foods that are causing them inflammation is carrying extra water weight. Depending on the age and size, this water weight can be a few ounces in a baby and up to 10 pounds in an adult. Losing this water weight quickly reveals your child's true level of malnourishment. Weight loss in itself isn't so harmful; rather, it's the malnourishment and maldigestion leading to it that are the bigger issue.

In the long run, it's important to make sure your child is eating enough and getting enough calories. Calories aren't everything, but they do matter. Children need plenty of protein and fat for growth, since those are the materials we're constructed from. They also need a source of starch, so don't overlook the winter squashes, cooked carrots, cooked beets, and fruit on grain-free diets. Make sure your child is eating nutrient-dense meals with a balanced amount of fat, protein, and carbs. Sneak in what he doesn't like however you can, to keep it balanced.

If gaining weight is a long-term issue and your doctor recommends adding more grains or starches, experiment with different types and amounts to see what might work for your child and still keep her on track to heal. Make sure your grains are properly prepared according to the Nourishing Traditions guidelines, if your child has digestive issues [see Resources].

Urinary tract or vaginal yeast infections

Even in children, these sometimes happen, particularly in girls. Avoid all fruit and honey, and keep them well-hydrated with meat stock and filtered water. Increase their probiotic capsules, if possible. Have them take baking soda baths each night. Then, apply homemade kefir (ideal) or yogurt (second choice) as a cream all over the vaginal area or groin.

Vomiting

If you suspect it's a blood sugar issue, mix up a few tablespoons of coconut oil with a small amount of honey and carry the jar around with you. Offer a teaspoon here and there to your child as your intuition tells you they need it, to help keep their blood sugar stable during the first couple weeks of the diet. I promise that they won't keep eating this forever. Refer to the Chapter 6 for more details.

If you feel like too much fat is the problem, refer to Chapter 7 for recommendations.

Watery diarrhea

When you start a new diet, your child might have a bout of diarrhea, even when it's something they've never experienced before, and especially if constipation is the norm for them. I don't worry over an instance of diarrhea or even a couple of days of loose stools. This is a natural cleansing reaction.

If diarrhea is your main symptom and primary reason for changing your child's diet, then you need to pay special attention to what helps and what triggers them. They might be triggered by FODMAPS foods (groups of foods containing specific types of carbohydrates), oxalate dumping, an allergen, or it may just be a detox reaction.

Whether diarrhea is common or a new thing for them, if they experience loose stools after trying a probiotic or fermented food, you can generally consider that a detox or die-off reaction. Beet kvass, for example, contains probiotics and stimulates the liver so it can cause both, and you'll need to adjust their "dose" accordingly.

Diarrhea is a cleansing reaction, because blood that's been circulating throughout the body (and liver) delivers toxins to the bowel wall, and as they cross through the wall into the lumen (open space) of the colon, they cause irritation and inflammation to the wall. The natural defense reaction of our intestinal tract is to pull salt and water into the bowel to cause diarrhea, in an attempt to move the toxins out of our body quickly.

In some people, diarrhea is combined with fecal compaction, which means the bowel is full of old, hard feces that are glued to the colon wall. The compacted feces produce toxins, causing the bowel to draw water and salt, resulting in loose stools. It might even come out in strange shapes like ribbons, due to squeezing past the hard masses. Even though your child may pass loose or soft stools every day, this is actually a combination of constipation and diarrhea. Unfortunately, passing the stool doesn't shift the compacted masses and doesn't completely empty the bowel.

Following a gut healing diet resolves this in the majority of kids over time. However, some kids still have fecal compaction after following a special diet for a year or longer, which can be confirmed with an x-ray. In these cases, a course of enemas or colonic hydrotherapy can be very helpful.

In order to heal watery diarrhea, it's essential to remove fiber from the diet, because it irritates the already inflamed intestines. Healing can't happen in the intestines without probiotic microbes, so be sure to include probiotic supplements or fermented foods.

Fermented dairy products, especially higher-protein kinds like yogurt and kefir, are very helpful in resolving diarrhea. I recommend introducing them right from the beginning, unless your child has an anaphylactic allergy. If they're sensitive to dairy, you can start with one teaspoon a day of whey dripped from homemade goat or camel's milk yogurt. These are the same recommendations I make to people who catch a tummy bug or traveler's diarrhea. When the diarrhea is over, go back to the foods you were eating before.

In times of profuse watery diarrhea, take all grains, vegetables, and fruit out of the diet. Have your child drink warm meat stock every hour with probiotic foods added to it. Serve them well-cooked gelatinous meats and add egg yolks gradually. Don't introduce vegetables of any kind until the diarrhea has calmed down. Contrary to popular belief, it's totally fine to go without vegetables for a short time.

Overcoming diarrhea requires patience and listening to the needs of your child's body as it heals itself in its own order. This means they won't be completely healed overnight, but the overall trend should be that they're getting better as the months go by. If their diarrhea isn't resolving at all within the first couple of weeks of following these suggestions, make an appointment with a practitioner who can help you dig a little deeper and test for pathogens and parasites.

CHAPTER 11: WHAT TO DO BEFORE YOU GIVE UP

As a Nutritional Therapy Practitioner, I'm completely passionate about seeing people succeed on healing diets. They are hard work and if you're putting in the effort and not seeing the results, you may wonder if it's time to throw in the towel and try something else.

First, go back and completely re-read your diet book to make sure you haven't overlooked or slacked off on a crucial component. These plans encompass so many changes that it's easy to forget about a couple of the recommendations. If you're not making any of those mistakes, what next? Some kids are very complex and you need to dig deeper. Here's the list of testing and next steps that I recommend.

Consult a Practitioner who specializes in the diet you're following

An experienced practitioner will be able to review what you've done so far and offer suggestions that you may have overlooked, or offer ideas based on the latest research. If you've been going it alone, or even if you've worked with a practitioner in the past, find someone with greater expertise. This could be somebody who's an expert in the diet itself, or it might be somebody who is an expert in your kids' specific health condition. There are often changes that need to be made to suit your child as an individual. Having somebody weigh in on a few adjustments can make all the difference in seeing results with any healing diet.

Try supplements

If you've followed your chosen diet's food list perfectly and you're still not seeing results, your child may be one who needs supplemental support. Especially if they still have digestive symptoms, consider giving digestive support supplements. Their body might very well need the kick-start that these supplements provide, in order to get to the next layer of healing. Digestive supplements include support for stomach acid, digestive enzymes, and fat digestion.

Food sensitivity and stool testing

Kids, especially when they're nonverbal, can be tricky little puzzles. If you're running into dead ends on the diet, it's time to find out more details from their body through testing. I recommend doing comprehensive stool testing at the same time as food sensitivity testing, because you need to address both tests together.

Comprehensive stool testing should tell you the amount of good and pathogenic bacteria present, along with any "weeds" that aren't pathogens, but need to be kept in check. You'll also want a test that looks for fungal overgrowth and parasites. In addition, look for markers that show digestive function, like if there's a need for digestive enzymes or fat digestion support, and look at markers of gut inflammation.

Food sensitivity testing (not just allergies, but sensitivities) performed at the same time will show you which foods are leading to reactions that cause inflammation in your kid at the moment. Remove those for three to six months, as indicated by the test you use.

As you address the stool testing with new probiotics, digestive support supplements, antibiotics, antifungals, or anti-parasitics, and remove any offending foods at the same time, their gut gets a break and can heal more quickly, allowing you to bring new foods in.

Nutrient testing

Nutrient testing through the blood, urine, or stool should be comprehensive and give you specific supplement recommendations to follow for three to six months. This alone can help show the holes in your child's nutrition (possibly related to genetic factors) and help resolve small, long-standing issues. Treat these new supplements like you would any new food and add them one at a time to look for any issues, like detox reactions.

Get genetic testing

In some cases, there are parts of any diet that aren't really helpful to your kid as an individual, because your child has a genetic factor working against them. This is a complex subject, so I won't talk about all the types of genetic variations that can cause issues. To give you a couple basic examples, they might have a gene that makes it difficult for them to process the sulfur in cruciferous vegetables. Or they might have a gene variation that makes it difficult for their liver to process certain vitamins, which hinders their detoxification. In these cases, certain foods that are supposed to be detoxifying and health-giving will actually make your kid feel kind of terrible. Figuring those things out with genetic testing can also help you alter any diet, to make it work for your kid and get them back on the path to healing. The cheapest genetic testing available is through 23andme.com [see Resources].

Just be aware that healing the gut comes first, and this is a later step in the journey.

Don't go back to crap!

If all has failed or you just don't think the diet works for you kid, don't give up everything and let your kid go back to a standard junk food diet. There are other healing philosophies out there that might suit your kid better, but *none of them contain processed foods*. Choose your next direction and dive in. Don't just throw out the whole concept of a healing diet.

CHAPTER 12: MY CHILD WON'T...

Every kid is different, and the foods they don't like or won't accept vary. If you've tried the methods in this book to get them eating in the first place, and you're struggling to get in one of the main healing foods or supplements that's required on their new diet, I have some tips for you.

Work through the ideas listed and let them inspire your own creativity. Don't give up—you will figure this out!

My child won't drink meat stock or broth...

This is the most common issue, and you're not alone.

- If your child is small, or open to taking broth "like medicine," give it to them in a syringe, so they don't have to taste it so much.

- Make sure your stock tastes good! Do you like it? Your kids don't like funky tasting stock either. Change up the herbs and seasonings to try different flavors. Try extra garlic, ginger, herbs, or curry paste, if allowed on your diet.

- Offer them stock from meat, poultry, fish, exotic meats, and other seafood. They might like one type and hate all the rest.

- Add a tiny amount to herbal tea, lemonade, or fresh pressed juice. Then, increase the ratio of stock over time.

- Cook all your meats and veggies in it so they are getting the drippings.

- Add a few drops to the sauerkraut juice or beet kvass to mask the flavor.

- Whisk some into a sauce like mustard, ketchup, or guacamole (or just pureed avocado).

- Add it to a smoothie.

- Let them drink it through a fun straw or sippy cup.

- Use it in a thick, blended veggie soup. Some kids don't like thinner soups or drinking broth straight.

- Add it to beaten eggs before you scramble them or turn them into a frittata.

- Reduce it down and make gravy (with nut flour if your diet is grain-free).

- Add a little to pancake batter.

- Add some to mashed potatoes or cauliflower.

- Add some to salad dressings.

- Use a little broth instead of water when you reheat leftovers on the stove.

- Use it as the liquid for stir-fry.

- Cook your lentils and beans in it.

- Sautee your meatballs or burgers in it.

- Turn it into an ice pop with some juice.

- Add it to juice or pureed fruit and make it into gelatin or a gummy snack.

- Try any of these suggestions with the fat skimmed off. You can work that in over time.

- Try any of these suggestions with a bland chicken feet stock.

Some stock is better than none. Find something that works, even if you're starting small.

My child won't drink water...

If your child is fasting from food, you must keep them hydrated. If they refuse plain water, here are some other options:

- Herbal teas like peppermint, chamomile, or ginger.

- Lemonade (see recipe in Chapter 5).

- Fresh pressed juices, like carrot juice.

My child won't drink juice…

- Play with the ratio of ingredients. Do they like it with more lemon juice, ginger, carrot, or a little green apple?

- Play with the colors. Some kids don't want green or brown juice but like it pink or red, so you can always add a little beet.

- Put it in a fun cup or let them sip it with a special straw.

- Try it as an ice pop.

- Make it into fruit gelatin (like Jell-o™) or gummy snacks.

Yes, you lose a bit of the nutrition in the last two options, but it's a place to start and some is better than none.

My child won't eat soups…

- Try pureed or "cream" soups.

- Try soup with chunky veggies.

- Try soup with pureed veggies and chunks of meat.

- Try offering them plain broth with boiled meat or meatballs, and veggies on the side.

- Still no? Try working things into a smoothie instead.

My child won't eat vegetables...

- Cauliflower and peeled cucumber or zucchini have the least noticeable tastes and are the easiest to sneak in.

- Mince or puree veggies and add them to ground meats, like in meatballs, meatloaf, or hamburgers.

- Try different combinations in blended soups with different herbs or seasonings to mask the flavors.

- Drench them with butter or cheese.

- Mince or puree them and add them to scrambled eggs.

- Make butternut squash or other veggie "fries."

- Puree some and add them to a more flavorful sauce like ketchup, mustard, gravy, or spaghetti sauce.

- Spiralize them into noodles and cover them with sauces.

- Juice them in tasty combinations.

- Take a look at your child's texture preferences and work within them.

- Have your child grow a couple of veggies in a garden, pick out foods to try at the farmer's market, or run them through the juicer. Getting them involved in the process of food prep and cooking makes them more likely to try something new.

My child won't eat chunky or hard textures...

- Try pureed meat and veggies in the soups.

- Get creative with smoothies, adding broth, veggie juice, avocado, chicken, or a little collagen powder for more protein.

- Try the purees in your own squeezable pouch if they don't like eating with utensils.

Work within your child's texture preferences for now, and make sure you're working *on* their texture preferences with other therapies as well.

My child won't eat purees or smoothie textures...

- Try chunky soups with veggies that are not too soft.

- Disassemble a soup and have them eat the meat and veggies on a plate.

- Make butternut squash or other veggie "fries" in the oven.

- Try the meats as meatballs or meatloaf.

- If they won't do runny egg yolks, scramble the egg yolks, even if they aren't trying the whites yet.

- Try juice as an ice pop or gummy snack.

Work within your child's texture preferences for now, and make sure you're working *on* their texture preferences with other therapies as well.

My child won't eat fish or seafood…

Don't let them miss all the trace minerals and essential fats from fish and seafood. Try these ideas:

- Add a small amount of fish stock to their chicken, beef, or other stocks. Start small and increase the ratio over time.

- Cook chunks of white fish in a chicken stock with lots of herbs and seasonings.

- Make fish sticks with almond or coconut flour breading.

- Find a shrimp or fish cake recipe, plus a dipping sauce for it.

- Mix ground seafood or fish into other ground meat and make burgers or meatballs.

- Expose them to different types of fish and seafood in different recipes, including those you don't like.

- Take them fishing, clamming, or crabbing. Being involved in procuring their own food can increase their interest in trying it.

My child won't eat avocado…

- Blend it into a smoothie.

- Make guacamole or other sauces that add different flavors.

- Puree some into a creamy soup.

My child won't eat eggs...

- Mix them into soups. The yolks will disappear and the whites become like egg drop soup if they're added in at the end.

- Blend them into smoothies.

- Bake them into pancakes and muffins.

- Use them to bind meatloaf and meatball.

- Mix the yolks into sauces like mustard, gravy, or dressings with olive oil and herbs.

CONCLUSION

Take a deep breath and imagine what it will feel like when your whole family is eating cheerfully.

The time you put into cooking is so worth it when your family is gathered together around a wholesome meal, sharing about their day.

Making a big food change with your picky eater isn't going to be easy at first, but the strategies and tips in this book will set you on the course for your dream life in the future. Instead of dinner being a stressful fight, you can breathe a sigh of relief as you serve your children nutritious foods that they'll eat happily every day.

The fact that you're here tells me you're ready to end picky eating and fulfill that peaceful dinner table fantasy.

Take action by mapping out the strategy for your family now. Then, tackle the preparation step-by-step, gaining confidence in your readiness to implement the diet change method you chose.

Your kids have already taught you that you're capable of handling so much more than you ever imagined.

So, yes, you *can* do this.

If you'd like to learn more and connect with a community of other parents who are ending picky eating, I invite you to join me at www.bodywisdomnutrition.com.

RESOURCES

Preface

My GAPS Diet Diary blog posts: http://bodywisdomnutrition.
com/my-gaps-diet-journey/

Dr. Natasha Campbell McBride can be found on the web at
www.gaps.me and www.doctor-natasha.com.

Chapter 1: How You Got a Picky Kid

Research on toxin exposure during pregnancy: https://www.
ewg.org/research/body-burden-pollution-newborns/detailed-
findings#.WlQOjN-nE2x

Chapter 2: Shape Your Mindset

Montessori recommendations for age-appropriate kitchen
tasks: www.flandersfamily.info/web/age-appropriate-chores-for-
children

Chapter 4: Get Prepared

How to reheat food without a microwave: www.gnowfglins.com/food-preparation/weekly-kitchen-tips/reheating-foods-without-a-microwave

Chapter 5: What to Expect as You Begin

Information on unconsciousness as a symptom of low blood sugar: www.diabetes.org/living-with-diabetes/treatment-and-care/blood-glucose-control/hypoglycemia-low-blood.html

Chapter 6: Anticipate Reactions

The Pulse Test book: www.soilandhealth.org/book/the-pulse-test

Find current supplement brand recommendations on my website: http://bodywisdomnutrition.com/picky-eater-approved/

Chapter 7: How to Know If You Need Supplements

Beet kvass recipe: www.bodywisdomnutrition.com/recipe-beet-kvass

Magnesium recommended daily intake: www.mayoclinic.org/drugs-supplements/magnesium-supplement-oral-route-parenteral-route/description/drg-20070730

Chapter 8: Detox Your Home

EWG skin deep database: http://www.ewg.org/skindeep/

EWG household cleaning database: www.ewg.org/guides/
cleaners-.Wfe2zohrw2w

Home Mold Identification: www.mycometrics.com

Chapter 10: Troubleshooting Issues

Histamine intolerance resource:. www.healinghistamine.com/

Salicylates and phenols food guide: www.salicylatesensitivity.
com/about/food-guide

Nourishing Traditions Cookbook, guidelines for soaking and
sprouting grains. Available on Amazon www.amzn.to/2gPTvib
(affiliate link)

Chapter 11: What to Do Before You Give Up

Genetic testing through 23andme.com: http://bit.
ly/23andmeBWN (Affiliate link)

CPSIA information can be obtained
at www.ICGtesting.com
Printed in the USA
LVOW03*1937190318
570348LV00015B/433/P